MY BIG FAT GREEK DIET

MY BIG FAT GREEK DIET

How a 467-Pound Physician Hit His Ideal Weight and How You Can Too

NICK YPHANTIDES, M.D.

WITH MIKE YORKEY

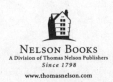

NELSON BOOKS
A Division of Thomas Nelson Publishers
Since 1798
www.thomasnelson.com

Published in Nashville, Tennessee, by Thomas Nelson, Inc.

Author is represented by the literary agency of Alive Communications, Inc., 7680 Goddard Street, Suite 200, Colorado Springs, CO 80920.

Scripture quotations noted NKJV are from THE NEW KING JAMES VERSION. Copyright © 1979, 1980, 1982, Thomas Nelson, Inc., Publishers.

Scripture quotations noted NLT are from the *Holy Bible,* New Living Translation, copyright © 1996. Used by permission of Tyndale House Publishers, Inc., Wheaton, Illinois 60189. All rights reserved.

Scripture quotations noted CEV are from THE CONTEMPORARY ENGLISH VERSION. © 1995 by the American Bible Society. Used by permission.

PUBLISHER'S NOTE: This book is intended for general health-care information only and is not intended to supplant medical advice, diagnosis, or treatment by a personal physician. Readers are urged to consult their physician before beginning any weight-loss program.

Library of Congress Cataloging-in-Publication Data

Yphantides, Nick.
   My big fat Greek diet : how a 467-pound physician hit his ideal weight and how you can too / Nick Yphantides with Mike Yorkey.
     p. cm.
   ISBN 0-7852-6025-0
   1. Weight loss. I. Yorkey, Mike. II. Title.
RM222.2Y695 2004
   613.2'5—dc22

                                       2004014404

Printed in the United States of America
04 05 06 07 08 QW 9 8 7 6 5 4 3

TO MY DESPINA

CONTENTS

INTRODUCTION

Is it true that you lost all this weight going to baseball games?" The inquiry came from Josh Valdez, the regional director of the U.S. Department of Health and Human Services. I met him while attending a White House conference on Faith-Based and Community Initiatives in my hometown of San Diego. As a family physician who has spent his entire professional life caring for the poor and indigent in the community health clinic system (I have never seen a patient with private medical insurance), I was keenly interested in how the medical community and the federal government could work together to meet the needs of those who've fallen through the holes of the nation's safety net.

"Well, it's not as simple as that," I said. "Going to the baseball games was a fun diversion while I drank protein shakes and exercised on the road."

"I've never met anybody who's lost as much weight as you have without having surgery," Josh commented.

"Neither have I," I replied. "I guess my story is fairly unusual. I spent eight months on the road, crisscrossing the country and taking in more than one hundred major-league baseball games at every American and National League ballpark. I didn't eat any solid food during my road trip. Instead, I drank two or three protein shakes a day."

"How much did you weigh when you started?" Josh asked.

"I can tell you the exact amount—467 pounds. I kept at it until I lost 270 pounds, which is the combined weight of *two* average-sized

American women standing five feet four inches and weighing 135 pounds."

I could tell Josh was intrigued by my story. "What are you doing for lunch?" he asked. "You do . . . eat, right?"

"Of course. I love to eat," I laughed. "I just don't eat like I used to."

"Good. I know this excellent family-run Mexican restaurant in Old Town. They have great posole," he said, referring to a meat stew containing pork and kernels of corn or hominy with all the trimmings—hot peppers, chopped onions, and diced chilies. "Want to join me?"

Josh didn't have to ask twice. Midway through our meal, as I entertained my new friend with anecdotes from my weight-loss baseball tour, he stopped me. "Nick, this is incredible. How would you like to come to Washington, D.C., to share your remarkable adventure?"

I nearly choked on my fresh corn tortilla. "Come to Washington? As in D.C.? Sure. Who would you like me to speak to?"

"We have a monthly meeting of the regional directors who report to Secretary of Health Tommy Thompson and the White House liaison to the Department of Health and Human Services, and we'd like to have you come and tell us how you lost the weight. Perhaps there's something we can learn from you," Josh said.

"When would you like me to come?" I asked with excitement rising in my voice.

"Let's see," he said, pulling out his calendar book. "How would Tuesday, April 1, sound? I'm thinking about one o'clock in the afternoon."

I nearly fell out of my chair when I heard Josh say April 1, not because I thought he could be pulling off an elaborate April Fools' joke, but because that date meant so much to me. You see, April 1, 2001, was the day my remarkable weight-loss story began.

MY CORE MESSAGE

What I told the DHHS regional directors that afternoon in our nation's capital forms the core message of this book—that you have to change your life before you can change your weight. I'm going to teach you how to do that through my Seven Pillars to Weight Loss and Maintenance, but in Part I of *My Big Fat Greek Diet*, I will tell you my story. In the past, I would have told you, "Do as I say, not as I do." Now I can humbly say, "Do as I say, and as I have done."

You see, I had reached a point in my midthirties where I desperately wanted to change my life. Eating had always been important in our ethnic family, but perhaps that's because I'm as Greek as homemade baklava. My father, George Yphantides (pronounced Eee-fahn-tee-dees), grew up in northern Greece near the base of Mount Olympus. He came to North America in the mid-1950s to attend college in Canada and then the United States. While in New Jersey, he met a wonderful American woman named Bernice Pfaff. They fell in love and were married.

Just over a year later, I—the firstborn of five children—arrived on the scene. When I was four years old, Dad moved his young family back to Greece, where we lived for nearly five years. While living in an Athens suburb, I was enrolled in grammar school, where, as the joke goes, everything was Greek to me.

When I was in the fifth grade, our family returned to the United States, resettling in New Jersey. I had to learn English all over again, but I had a good ear and a good aptitude for schoolwork. I was allowed to skip two grades during my school years, so when I graduated from Tenafly High School in New Jersey, I was a peach-fuzzed and pudgy sixteen-year-old who weighed thirty or forty pounds more than an average kid my age.

I headed west for college, attending Azusa Pacific University in Southern California, where I graduated three and a half years later with plans to become a doctor. There was no doubt I was getting heavy since I weighed 280 pounds. Dad and Mom had always encouraged me to follow my dreams, and my dream was to care for the sick and infirm. Practicing medicine among those who needed it most greatly appealed to me.

While applying to medical school, I earned a master's degree in public health from Loma Linda University. Then the good news arrived in the mailbox: The University of California at San Diego (UCSD) School of Medicine had accepted my application, and when I graduated five years later at the age of twenty-six, I was one of the youngest physicians in a class of 126. A one-year internship in family practice, and *voilà:* At age twenty-seven, I hung my shingle at the Escondido Community Health Center, located thirty miles northeast of San Diego.

It was in medical school that I became morbidly obese, which is medically defined as being at least one hundred pounds overweight. I was now over three hundred pounds, and I couldn't stop eating, especially since I "rewarded" myself for studying so hard. For instance, when I pulled all-nighters during finals week, I fortified my body with Ding-Dongs and Rocky Road ice cream and late-night raids of the refrigerator. During interminable forty-hour shifts as an intern, I kept my energy up and my eyes open with periodic visits to the hospital canteen, where invariably someone had set out a plate of sweets to be shared by the attending staff.

When I entered the public health arena as a family physician, I could be best described as "corpulent." I can't tell you how much I weighed because I had stopped weighing myself. I was like a runaway train, adding pounds each month. To compensate, I threw myself into my work with my patients, putting in ninety-hour weeks following my promotion to medical director of the Escondido Community Health Center. I loved my work because I was drawn to caring for the less fortunate, of which there were plenty in this working-class city surrounded by avocado trees and orange groves. Many of my patients were Hispanics—some undocumented, some not—who had found themselves outside "the system." They and their families did not have health insurance, and thus they were funneled toward public health programs.

My expanding girth actually became an occupational blessing: My patients viewed me as a larger-than-life advocate for the poor, the big man with a big heart who cared for his community in a big way. Overweight patients *loved* me because they knew they would receive tea and sympathy from someone who also shopped at Mr. Big and Tall. From a doctor's perspective, I was always gracious with people who struggled with their weight. More than a few times, I can remember saying with a glint in my eye, "Do as I say, not as I do."

My weight continued to balloon as I turned thirty. When I began experiencing declining health and a host of unusual symptoms, however, I made an appointment to see a specialist. A week later, I learned the bad news: I had testicular cancer. This type of cancer is rare, but if a man in his thirties is diagnosed with cancer, it's likely to be testicular. As with all cancers, early diagnosis makes all the difference in the world.

I'm not going to sugarcoat this—I was scared. The surgical excision of my right testicle and aggressive radiation during a twelve-week period saved my life—and caused some soul-searching. The way I saw things, I had dodged the cancer bullet, but there was another round in the chamber: My gargantuan weight had to be causing incredible amounts of stress on my organs—heart, lungs, and liver—as well as my skeletal frame. I wondered how much stress I was putting on my knees, which were bearing such a severe load.

Cancer forced me to face my mortality, and I was sure that each bite of a double-deluxe bacon cheeseburger brought me one swallow closer to the grave. Something needed to be done because I was in the throes of despair regarding my health, my physical limitations, the constant awareness of the special accommodations I needed, and the harsh, judgmental criticism I received from the general public.

For example, when I awoke each morning, the severe joint pain in my knees was so bad that I could barely shuffle my way to the bathroom. My ankles groaned in protest all day long—but I didn't want to stop playing on my church softball team, though I knew I would suffer for days after each game. I played first base—a position that didn't demand much movement—and I was a pretty good hitter.

No matter how many "gappers" I hit into the outfield alleys, though, I could never turn any of my long hits into doubles. When I safely reached first base, I knew I couldn't run the bases, so I requested a pinch runner. Even though I could get back into the game under our free substitution rules, I felt humiliated each time I replaced myself with a fitter teammate to run the base paths. But that was nothing compared to the razzing I got from the other bench the time I lined a base hit over the shortstop's head only to be thrown out at first base by the left fielder!

My life was inconvenienced in other ways. When I went out to eat, I dreaded walking into a new restaurant. Where was I going to sit? I couldn't slide into a booth, nor could I wedge myself into any chairs with armrests. I scrounged up a sturdy chair without armrests. One time, I wedged myself into a plastic patio chair at a Mexican restaurant. Midway through the meal, the chair split in two, and I fell in a heap. Another embarrassing episode. When the waiter arrived to help me off the floor, I claimed the chair was already cracked so I wouldn't have to pay for it.

I didn't accept rides with well-meaning friends unless I was *sure* they drove a big SUV like I did. I needed the extra room as my waistline expanded. Throughout my adult years, I drove a succession of oversized vehicles—a Bronco, an Explorer, and an Expedition—because they were large enough for me to squeeze in behind the wheel. (The seat belt was never big enough for me to cinch around my body, however.)

Flying was even worse. I booked uncrowded red-eye flights whenever I traveled by air, but I'll never forget the time I had to fly from San Diego to Albuquerque for a medical conference. Southwest Airlines had the only nonstop—and the cheapest fare—so I booked a morning flight. I ran late that day and was handed a "C" boarding pass by the gate agent. That meant I would be among the last to board, and Southwest does not assign seats.

I squeezed myself down the narrow aisle with a deep sense of dread. My fondest wish was to find two small kids occupying a three-seat row on the 737, but some dreams weren't meant to come true. The reality that morning was an open middle seat between a man on the window and a middle-aged woman on the aisle.

When I approached that row, I could tell by the woman's look that she had received some bad news—like a death in the family.

"Excuse me," I offered, and she reluctantly stepped out of her seat so I could take the middle seat. I tried to sit down between the two armrests, but each armrest dug into my thighs. The more I pushed, the more it hurt.

"Would you mind if I brought this armrest up?" I wanly asked. Both of us understood the implication of my request: I would be spilling some of my excess poundage into her "space."

"Actually, I would mind," she said as she continued standing in the aisle.

An alert flight attendant sized up the situation. "Let me see if I can help you," she offered.

Two rows behind us, the flight attendant spotted a mother sitting in the window seat with a three-year-old occupying the middle seat and a nine-year-old boy on the aisle.

I turned my head and watched the flight attendant lean over to the mother and whisper something. The mother looked at me. With a pitying sigh, she nodded yes.

"We're going to switch you with the young boy," the Southwest flight attendant announced. As I stood up to make the move, she whispered, "Next time, sir, you need to buy two seats."

I gulped down another heavy helping of humiliation as everyone in that section of the plane watched me move from one row to another. Indignities like that happened continually to me—like the occasion when I escorted several out-of-town relatives to Tijuana so they could get a taste of Mexico. Tijuana's main drag is called Avenue Revolution, a beehive of buying and selling as a succession of shops and street vendors vie for the *Yanqui* dollar.

The street vendors were on us like mosquitoes that day, and as we strode past them, they kept up a steady chatter inviting us to buy their wares. One vendor with several dozen leather belts draped across one arm approached us and said in English, "Belts—I have belts for sale."

"No thank you," I said on behalf of everyone.

The vendor eyed me. "But we have them in your size, sir."

"No thank you," I repeated, anxious to keep moving and not to engage him in conversation.

We had walked several steps when I heard him say, "We even have them in *vaca gorda* size."

I understood what he said: He had belts big enough for a fat cow. I spun on my heels. I recognized the phrase because I spoke Spanish every day at the community health clinic where I practiced.

"Quien dices vaca gorda?" I demanded in Spanish. (Who are you calling a fat cow?)

"Lo siento, señor," the vendor replied, holding up his palms as fifteen of his buddies burst out in laughter. My face turned red, and I had suffered yet another humiliation.

My obesity also affected my social life. I had a very short romantic "rap sheet" as I was deemed unworthy and undesirable in the eyes of most women. I didn't like the rejection I felt after being turned down for a date. It was painful not to be able to get a date with women I found attractive. It was often obvious that they were repulsed by my size. Some friends tried to match me up with significantly overweight women, assuming that our ideal date would be sitting on a couch and sharing a half-gallon carton of cookie dough ice cream. Then again, I wasn't any great catch. My obesity and decreased life expectancy had to be legitimate concerns to any woman thinking long term. Who would want me to be the father of her children, only to leave her a widow with children to raise on her own fifteen or twenty years later?

The weight of dealing with my obesity sapped my morale. I was tired of dressing in XXXXL T-shirts and tent-sized gym pants, tired of gawkers staring at my monstrous midsection when I passed through the buffet line balancing two plates heaped high with food. What lay ahead was a future filled with high blood pressure, high cholesterol, debilitating diabetes—and premature death—unless I made some radical lifestyle changes and lost a ton of weight.

I was ready to change my life.

MAKING A GAME PLAN

On April 1, 2000 (yes, April Fools' again), I notified the Escondido Community Health Center that in one year, I would be stepping down as medical director and leaving my clinical practice. This was no April Fools' Day joke. I knew that I would need to take time off while I concentrated on losing so much weight. Monumental problems demand monumental solutions! Fortunately, I was not married and could refinance my home and take out equity to cover the cost of my upcoming adventure. I figured it would cost me more than $50,000 to step away from work, on top of my lost salary. I still had bills to pay, including medical school loans and a mortgage. I understand that few people can step away from work for a year—and somehow afford to do so, but, by the grace of God, I could. I made a significant financial sacrifice and put my economic and physical health future on the line.

I formulated a game plan. First, I decided to take an unconventional approach in addressing my personal health needs. Since I wasn't going to work, I needed something to do—a distraction to keep my mind off being so hungry. The thought came to me to combine doing something I totally enjoyed while doing something good for my health. Since I was a huge baseball fan (literally and figuratively), I could travel around the country watching baseball games in every major-league ballpark during a single baseball season—the ultimate pilgrimage for any baseball nut. As for losing weight, I decided to embark on a liquid fast—drinking a protein supplement offering just 800 calories a day. This would be a very aggressive diet since I calculated that I had been consuming an average of 5,600 calories a day up till then. (I'll be talking about liquid diets in detail in Chapter 13.)

Throughout this book, you'll read more about the remarkable transformation I experienced during my baseball tour of America *and* learn about "Dr. Nick's Seven Pillars," which are my key principles for weight reduction and maintenance. My hope and desire is that my story and these Seven Pillars will inspire you to lose weight as well as equip you with the tools you'll need to undergo your own transformation. Keep in mind that it's important to implement the Seven Pillars as a whole rather than piecemeal. You should also be sure to seek medical help and supervision prior to leaping into a life-changing transformation. As you think about how to go about this, you can use my Web site—www.healthsteward.com—as a clearinghouse of information.

Meanwhile, if you're holding this book because you're overweight—or know a family member who's struggling with his or her weight—then you've come to the right place for advice on how to lose weight. America has an obesity problem the likes of which this country—or any civilized nation—has never seen before. From early morning until midnight, we are awash in breakfast burritos, lunchtime burgers, and barrels of extra-crispy fried chicken for dinner. Pop a movie into the DVD player, and before you know it, we're ordering a late-night thick-crust, extra-cheese, all-meat pizza. Our collective propensity for eating high-fat, high-calorie food is producing a land of lard and a country of couch potatoes.

Today, 65 percent of U.S. adults are classified as overweight by the Centers for Disease Control—nearly two-thirds of us! Compare this sobering statistic to twenty years ago, when less than half of all (46 percent) Americans were considered overweight. What's even more astounding is that half of all overweight people (or one-third of the adult American population) can be considered obese, meaning that they weigh at least fifty pounds over their ideal body weight.

In 2002, the Internal Revenue Service classified obesity as a disease and began allowing taxpayers to take medical deductions for expenses related to treatment—fitness trainers, gastric bypass surgery, and commercial weight-loss programs like Jenny Craig. The population boom of fat people has also sparked a gold rush for companies promising to make life even more comfy and cushy for the obese. Overweightpeople.com, for instance, will sell you everything from custom-made bicycles for riders up to six hundred pounds to airline seat-belt extenders to extra-wide umbrellas to extra-long shoehorns.

Major car manufacturers and furniture and supply companies have also responded to the bloating of America by:

- widening seats in trucks and SUVs
- extending seat belts so that obese people aren't pinched
- producing desk chairs that are five inches wider and will support five hundred pounds

- introducing five-hundred-pound-capacity recliner chairs that lift and tilt forward so that obese people can get in and out of them more easily
- selling heavy-duty toilets, wheelchairs, and patient hoists to hospitals

Perhaps the last time you shopped for a car, you chose a more expensive SUV over a more sporty two-door because you could fit behind the wheel of the Suburban but not the Miata. Perhaps the last time you showed up at an airline ticket counter, you were told to buy a second seat the next time around, as I was told by Southwest Airlines. Perhaps the last time you shopped for clothes, you couldn't stand the thought of buying another muumuu and boring plus-size clothes produced for the "full-figure" market. Perhaps you've been one hundred pounds overweight since high school, and it's starting to take a toll on your joints.

If you're ready to do something about your excess weight, I can't guarantee that you'll be successful after you read this book, but I can guarantee that you'll be inspired and have the tools to finally do something. In Part I of this book, I will share the story of how I once weighed 467 pounds before taking a nine-month sabbatical from work and from eating solid food. In Part II, I will shift gears and share how you can lose weight by following my Seven Pillars of Weight Loss and Maintenance. Finally, in Part III, I will explain how to order the right items in fast-food restaurants; advise parents of obese children on what they can do to help their kids become healthier; and give some doctorly advice on the pros and cons of the latest development in weight loss— gastric bypass surgery, also known as "stomach stapling."

Let me close this introduction by telling you that as a physician and as a cancer survivor, if you don't have your health, you don't have anything. Being overweight or obese is unhealthy, and it will take years off your life span. Please, please do something while there's still time.

You won't regret it. If you're successful in slimming down, then you'll experience a big fat Greek miracle.

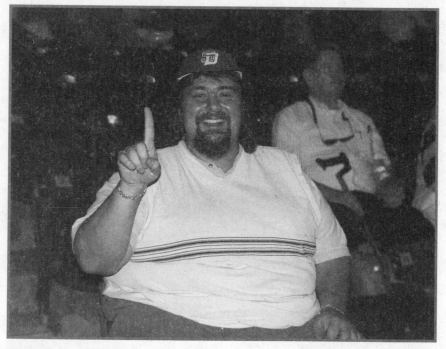

When I sat at San Diego Padre baseball games, I made sure I had an aisle seat.

PART I

MY **BIG FAT GREEK DIET**

THE PARABLE OF MY LIFE

CHAPTER 1

THE LAST SUPPER

March 31, 2001
San Diego, California

I strode into the cherrywood-paneled and well-appointed foyer of the Ruth's Chris Steak House with my father and two younger brothers, John and Phil, close behind me. An attractive hostess in a black sleeveless dress stood sentry behind a lectern.

"May I help you?" she offered with a cheery smile.

"Yes, we have reservations for tonight, party of four. The reservation should be under Dr. Nick." I had long given up making dinner reservations with a last name like Yphantides.

"Let's see . . . Oh, here you are," she said as she pulled four menus from their eye-level perch. "If you will follow me."

As our foursome fell in behind her and filed into the deco-motifed dining room, a waiter hefting a large silver tray passed by. A half dozen filets, rib eyes, and New York strips—broiled in pan-seared butter— sizzled in their juices, creating a succulent aroma that threatened to make me feel light-headed. I soldiered on, knowing that we could order several Ruth's Chris appetizers within minutes after being seated in this old-style steak house, and that would sate my hunger pains until the real food came along.

"Doesn't the menu look amazing, Dad?" I said as I began flipping through the delectable offerings on the leather-bound carte du jour.

"It sure does, son," he replied. "I'm so glad we came here for your last meal."

My last meal. I felt like a condemned man, all right. If everything went according to plan, this Saturday evening, March 31, 2001, would be the last time I would eat solid food for the next eight months. The following day—and it would be no April Fools' joke—I planned to drink only protein shakes until I became half the man I used to be.

I needed to lose weight. I was fat—flabby, portly, plump, stout, chubby, obese—whatever you want to call it. I wasn't exactly sure how much I weighed because the medical-quality scale that I used to weigh myself stopped at 350 pounds. All I knew was that when I stepped onto the scale, the needle shot toward the 350 mark, so I assumed that my weight had to be a bit north of 350 pounds. That's why, after a year of planning, I finally decided to do something about it. I was leaving my job at the Escondido Community Health Center and embarking on a weight-reducing odyssey that would take me to all fifty U.S. states and to every major-league baseball park in the country.

I planned to treat myself to more than one hundred American

League and National League baseball games since I could no longer indulge myself with food. Along the way, I would shed weight like a musk ox sheds its fur coat after a long winter. My goal: Lose 150 pounds through an aggressive weight-loss regimen of drinking protein supplement drinks totaling 800 calories a day.

The evening at Ruth's Chris to celebrate the start of the trip was actually my idea, but that's because I'm Greek and I love festive occasions. Growing up in the Hellenic culture taught me the importance of memorializing certain moments of my existence with events of special significance. American translation: Any time is a good time to party. But hey, I'm Greek, and that's the way life is meant to be lived, which is why I love celebrating national holidays and creating a few of my own. For our gastronomical foray to Ruth's Chris Steak House, I dubbed this evening "The Last Supper," which seemed appropriate because it would be my last meal of solid food for a long, long time.

I just wished more family members could have joined us since Greek frivolity involves *all* the family. My dear mother, Bernice, the matronly pillar of support for our family, would have loved to have been part of this special meal. Unfortunately, she, along with my brother Paul, my sister Pauline, and one sister-in-law, Heather, had traveled cross-country for *another* family event—the bridal shower of my future sister-in-law, Eleni. She would be marrying my younger brother, Paul, in Boston on Memorial Day Weekend, and I planned to be there during my weight-loss sabbatical. This was a big fat Greek wedding that I would not miss.

Dad, the patriarch of the family, did not make the trip back east for the bridal shower since he would be the navigator at the beginning of my cross-country trip. This would be a guys' night out, a time for the Yphantides men to blow the doors off one of the best eateries in San Diego—Ruth's Chris Steak House. As we were seated in our upholstered chairs that evening, a thick orange sun moved quickly toward the Pacific horizon in the West.

"And what may I start you gentlemen off with tonight?" inquired our waiter, dressed in a starched white shirt, thin black tie, and coal-black pants. He held a pad and a pencil in his hands, and for the next three hours, we nearly gave him writer's cramp.

One thing I knew: We would not be hurried on such a special evening. "I think we would like to start with some appetizers," I said, and I placed an order for my two favorites—the Barbecued Shrimp and the Mushrooms Stuffed with Crabmeat. My dad and brothers each ordered something off the appetizer page, including cold shrimp swimming in a Creole rémoulade sauce and fresh broccoli buried beneath an avalanche of melted cheddar cheese.

Our family has always enjoyed eating. Phil, thirty years old and weighing 230 pounds, was packing an extra thirty or forty pounds on his six-foot frame—weight that he had gained since his marriage to Betsy, who is a tremendous cook in her own right. John, a year older and also a six-footer, was in better shape. He was probably packing an extra ten or fifteen pounds around his midsection. Dad, a barrel-chested sixty-seven-year-old with a Michelin tire midriff, weighed 210 pounds on his five-foot, six-inch frame, but he had earned the right to enjoy the fruits of his labors.

Now that our first-wave assault of Ruth's Chris was under way, I turned my attention to the prize: the meat entrée and side dishes. A visitor to our table interrupted my concentration.

"Excuse me, but are you the guy in the newspaper who's going on the cross-country adventure to lose weight?" asked a trim man who was dressed well and looked to be in his early thirties.

He must have seen the North County Times *front-page feature on me in last Sunday's edition,* I thought with a hint of pride. The local media had latched on to my story, and my upcoming lose-weight-while-watching-baseball-games trip was the subject of numerous newspaper accounts and TV features in the San Diego area.

"Yes, that would be me," I said as I pushed myself out of the chair. "Hi, I'm Nick Yphantides. And you are—"

"Niece, George Niece. I'm really impressed with what you're going to try to do—lose all this weight while traveling around the country visiting ballparks. I mean, that's just amazing. I just want you to know that I clipped your story and stuck it to the poster board over my desk. You really are an inspiration to me."

Suddenly, I felt sick to my stomach. As this very nice fellow, George Niece, continued to shower me with verbal accolades regarding my courageous effort to lose weight, it struck me that I was about to gorge myself with rich food in an all-out food frenzy the likes of which I had probably never experienced. The thought that I would be willingly participating in a food orgy on the eve of a so-called "courageous" attempt to lose a massive amount of weight made me feel queasy.

I'm going to be honest here: I didn't feel queasy for long. After George departed, I shrugged off those ambivalent feelings when our half dozen appetizers arrived with a flourish and were set before our hungry eyes.

Tonight's meal would be the last time I would chew savory and succulent food for a long time, and I would celebrate that event in going-out-in-glory style. My evening at Ruth's Chris would be the pinnacle of thirty-five years of gluttony in one culinary experience, a no-holds-barred explosion of decadence. I truly believed that life's richest moments were meant to be celebrated with the mouth, tongue, and stomach.

For the next few hours, food spilled off our table. This was a voracious orgy on the order of King Arthur's Court, with plate after plate of delicious food eaten slowly and with purpose by myself and my father and my brothers. The bill would come to well over $300, but there would be nothing holding me back.

What did I order? The question would be better asked: *What didn't I order?* I mentioned the appetizers, which we shared, but our waiter couldn't keep the freshly baked bread and ceramic butter tubs coming quickly enough until the rest of the food came out in waves. I began with the Lettuce Wedge, a crisp wedge of iceberg lettuce with all the trimmings. Since Ruth's Chris was a classic meat-and-potatoes restaurant, I ordered three different potato dishes—au gratin; mashed with a hint of roasted garlic; and lyonnaise style, sautéed with onions—to accompany my *pièce de résistance,* the porterhouse strip *for two!* The cost for just the steak was $69, but this would be my special indulgence.

The waiter, to his credit, didn't raise an eyebrow. He probably sized up the situation and knew better than to ask me with whom I would be sharing my forty-ounce steak. Oh, and there was another thing. I asked the waiter, "Could you cook my steak in extra butter?"

"No problem, sir."

You may wonder if I was up to the task of eating two and half pounds of ultrarich and densely marbled USDA prime steak that evening. I was. For the better part of an hour, I savored the juicy, tasty steak at a relaxing pace. I wasn't in a hurry, although I joked with my family that we were losing one hour of eating time since daylight saving time started the next morning. I will confess that I had no problem polishing off my porterhouse steak for two, all my potato sides, plus what other food I could forage from our table, which, as you can imagine, was covered with appetizers, side dishes, and more baked bread. I ate until I thought food would come out my ears.

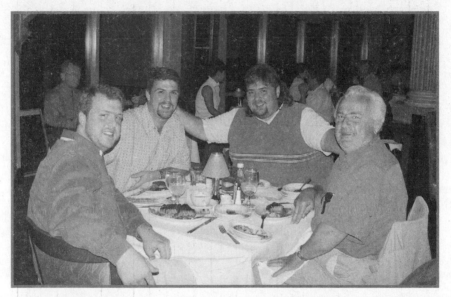

I celebrated "The Last Supper" at Ruth's Chris Steak House with my brothers Phil and John and my father, George, by having a no-holds-barred food orgy.

But I still had room for dessert. Make that two! I ordered a piece of cheesecake and a slice of banana cream pie, and I would not be sharing these desserts with my family—they could order their own, which they did.

I will never forget my last bite of real food before the start of my trip. It would be one that I would fantasize about as my brain screamed out for something more than another boring protein shake.

I looked at my second helping of dessert—a defenseless banana cream pie. As my father and brothers looked on, I heaped the final piece of banana cream pie onto my fork, took one last longing look as if to say good-bye to real food, and stuffed it into my mouth. Then I let the sugary dessert rest on my tongue. I did not chew, and I did not swallow. I sat back in my chair, closed my eyes, and leaned my head back to relish the sybaritic moment as the banana cream pie began to melt in the digestive juices produced by my overworked salivary glands.

My desire was to savor this last bit of sweet dessert for as long as I could and let it slowly dissolve down my gullet. When the last of the banana cream pie had washed down my esophagus, I opened my eyes and said, "It is finished."

One life had just ended.

A new life was about to begin.

CHAPTER TWO

WEIGH OVER
THE SCALE

Sunday, April 1
Escondido, California

I certainly woke up in a groggy state on the morning after the Ruth's Chris glut-fest. I was experiencing the lingering effects of FES—food engorgement syndrome. My binge overeating had to be the epicurean equivalent of a food hangover.

I glanced at my alarm clock. The red numerals stated 7:42 in the morning, the first day of the rest of my life without overeating. Time for a gut check. Was I hungry? No, I still felt completely sated from the evening before. Then I remembered that I hadn't even brushed my teeth before I went to bed because I hadn't wanted to cleanse my palate from the taste of food.

I couldn't believe that nearly two years of planning had come to this moment, the start of my weight-loss journey. I felt a manic sense of excitement and liberation, a nervous but euphoric feeling that something good would happen over the next eight months. The irony of beginning down this long road on April Fools' Day was inescapable. I had been a fool for allowing myself to get to this point, but I knew I would be a bigger fool if I failed to do anything about it.

Only Dad and I were home that morning, but my father was still sleeping off the Last Supper. I dragged myself out of bed and donned a bathrobe that barely covered my folds of flesh. When I walked into our living room, my younger brother Phil, who lived next door, had just come over. He had a cup of morning coffee in his hand.

"How are you feeling?" he asked.

"Kind of like a young kid on Christmas morning excited about unwrapping his presents, but I'm also anxious about what's underneath the gift wrap and inside the cardboard box," I said.

"Well, are you ready to get started?"

"Yeah," I said. I knew where this was going.

The day before, I had purchased a weight scale from a medical supply store identical to the one I already owned. Both scales stopped at 350 pounds. For the last few months, I had been stepping on one scale and watching the red needle *boing* to 350 pounds like a top-fuel dragster leaving the starting line. Since the arrow couldn't go past 350 pounds, however, I simply figured that I weighed 350-plus pounds. What the "plus" amounted to was an open-ended question. That's why, on Day One of my weight-loss journey, Phil and I would determine how much I really weighed once and for all. Then I would know how much weight I would officially have to lose.

There was another agenda as well. I wanted Phil, also a family physician, to medically supervise the weigh-in and provide photo documentation—take the "before" shots with a camera. I had also asked him to medically oversee my diet from start to finish because I had chosen an aggressive weight-loss plan that required a doctor's supervision. Having Phil on board would help keep me accountable as well.

My brother set the twin identical scales before me in the middle of our living room, then cleared his throat. I took that as my cue to disrobe. Wearing nothing more than a wan smile, I placed one foot on each scale. I had to lean over my bulging abdomen to see the readout, but contrary to what others say about fat people, I could see my feet. This time the red arrows each settled on the same number: $233\frac{1}{2}$ pounds. I started to do the math in my head. *Let's see . . . holy cow, that's 467 pounds!*

"Listen, Phil, this can't be right. I weigh closer to 350. There's no way I weigh 467 pounds."

Phil had performed the simple arithmetic as well. "Step on the scale again," he ordered.

I stepped off and then back on the two scales. The red arrows settled at $233\frac{1}{2}$ again.

I refused to believe what I was seeing. "Something's gotta be wrong here," I said as I stepped off and on the scale a third time, a fourth time, and a fifth time. That's when the truth hit me like a punch to the midsection—*you weigh 467 pounds!* What was left in my stomach from Ruth's Chris Steak House nearly wound up on the two scales. I felt nauseated with disgust.

"Lean to the left," my brother directed. I put more weight on my left foot, which moved the red needle to 269 pounds. The scale under my right foot now read 198 pounds. "Still 467," said Phil. When I leaned to the right, we received the same result when we added the two numbers together: 467 pounds.

I stepped off the scales and braced myself against the wall. This could not be! The reality hit me like a bucket of ice-cold water splashed in my face. Yes, I knew I was overweight, but anyone who weighed 467 pounds was a slob—a tub of lard, a mound of mush, and a gargantuan excuse for a human being. I also felt as though I was a liar because I had been telling everybody—including the San Diego media—that I weighed 350 pounds, give or take a few, *wink, wink*. Now I weighed 117 pounds more, which meant that my estimate was off by an entire gymnast!

Another thought depressed me. All along, I had been planning to lose 120 pounds on my weight-loss trip, since I weighed 350, right? Now the bar had been raised to what—220 pounds to lose? That seemed an impossible achievement.

I think my brother was in shock, too, because he wasn't saying much. The knot in my throat was such that I could not speak a word. "Let's do the pictures," he said, as if to take our minds off the weighty revelation.

"The camera's over there." I pointed to the fancy new Canon digital camera I had just purchased for the trip.

I stood in the middle of the living room while Phil proceeded to take a dozen pictures of my bloated, naked body from every angle imaginable. A sense of utter shame and embarrassment washed over me as Phil documented what twenty-five years of overeating and a lack of exercise had done to my body. Though the idea to take pictures was self-imposed, I felt violated and utterly devastated for letting myself get to this pathetic point. When the last flash picture had been taken, I began to cry. The lone solace was that since we were using a digital camera, we didn't have to take the roll of film to a local one-hour photo store to be developed, where the employees could pass around the humiliating pictures and laugh at me.

I hung my head as I walked toward the bathroom. I hoped that a shower would lift my spirits, and it did. Tears mixed with soapy water flowed freely. As the hot water cascaded over my now-certified 467-pound body, my shame turned to determination. As God was my witness, I would lose my excess weight once and for all.

PACKING UP

The rest of the day was more chaotic: a rumble-jumble of errands, shopping for drinks (notice that I didn't say food), paying bills, and packing up the 1990 Chevy conversion van that would be my home away from home for the next eight months. I loaded up the van with two dozen two-liter bottles of Diet Coke, Diet Mountain Dew, Diet Snapple Ice Teas, and Diet Orange Crush. These no-calorie drinks would serve as the liquid fortifier of the protein shakes I would be drinking twice a day to give me sustenance.

Packing up the van was easy since there wasn't any food to stow. (My father, who would be accompanying me periodically during the trip, did not want to eat in front of me, which is why we didn't bother taking along any regular food. Out of sight, out of mind was his thinking.) I also took along a new laptop computer and a "vanwarming" present: a road atlas that came with a helpful CD containing software that would direct me anywhere in the fifty United States.

How I came to purchase the Chevy conversion van was nothing short of miraculous. I had been looking for some type of used conversion van that didn't have too many miles or too big a price tag. My dad was driving through the neighborhood one day when he spotted a 1990 Chevy conversion van with a "For Sale" sign in the window.

Two things drew me to the van. First, it was clean and in great shape with no dents, but even better, the van had only thirty-seven thousand miles on it. When I asked why so few miles over eleven years of driving, I expected the owner to tell me that he drove it only to church on Sunday. Instead, he volunteered that he used the van to drive to a nearby shelter for battered women and children, where he gave them free haircuts in the van's "living room." I liked his altruism, so I purchased the van.

Then another interesting thing happened when the media began asking about my upcoming baseball trip. "How are you going to get around?" they asked.

"With this used conversion van I bought," I replied as I kicked the tires.

"You have a name for this vehicle?" one scribe asked.

I hadn't thought about naming a car before, but in a moment of inspiration, I said, "Yeah, it's called the USS *Spirit of Reduction*."

Thus, my Chevy van had been christened, and the catchy name USS *Spirit of Reduction* stuck with the media and with me. I liked how my new van was decked out. It came with a small kitchen and refrigerator, plus a table and couch; the latter converted into a bed. The other sleeping quarter was a loft bed above the driver's and front passenger seats, but I couldn't fit into that. My father couldn't climb into the loft bed because of his bad knees, so we ended up using the loft bed as a storage compartment.

The other major storage area was in the back of the conversion van, which was home to a toilet and two pantry closets. I stuffed the left pantry with packets of chocolate protein shake and the right pantry with vanilla packets. I wasn't taking much in the way of clothes. In fact, my wardrobe was built around one of the most thoughtful gifts I received prior to the trip. Brad and Amy Thomas, next-door neighbors who owned a silk-screening business, made me twenty-five T-shirts with "Dr. Nick's Stadium Tour" inscribed across the front in an L.A. Dodgers-like script. On the back of each T-shirt was my trip motto: "Taking a Swing at Weight Loss."

Brad and Amy put their faith in me that I would lose the weight. They gave me five sets of T-shirts (each set had a white, beige, blue, red, and gray shirt) in the following sizes:

- five shirts in XXXXL
- five shirts in XXXL
- five shirts in XXL
- five shirts in XL
- five shirts in L

These were the shirts that I would be wearing day in and day out for the next eight months. The rest of my wardrobe consisted of a black sweater (oversized, of course), gray sweatpants with a drawstring that I could cinch around my sixty-inch waist, and a pair of Nike sneakers that I purchased at Marshall's—12$^{1}/_{2}$, extra wide.

The lingering daylight—this was the first day of daylight saving time—was appreciated as I finished packing the van for our long road trip. I hadn't eaten all day or felt hungry, for which I was thankful. The hustle-bustle of last-minute packing had distracted me. As the day turned into evening, I needed some nourishment, so at 9 p.m., I fired up the blender for the first time. I mixed sixteen ounces of cold Diet Orange Crush and a vanilla protein shake packet and gulped it down.

The taste—kind of like an orange cream Popsicle—wasn't too bad. A half hour later, I was still hungry, so I made a second protein shake. This time, I mixed a Diet A&W Root Beer with a vanilla packet. Yummy! It tasted just like a root beer float.

Maybe I could get used to these shakes, I thought. Then again, I didn't have a choice.

Monday, April 2
Los Angeles

Play ball! Today was Opening Day of the 2001 Major League Baseball season across America, and my father and I planned to hit the road running by attending our first game at Chavez Ravine, home of the Los Angeles Dodgers.

The family members who were not back in Boston gathered at the family compound on Titan Court. Betsy—Phil's wife—brought along my little nephew Josiah, who had just turned six months of age.

Betsy carried her son to me. "Little Joey," she said, using his nickname, "was wondering if Uncle Nick could feed him his first solid food."

I melted. "Oh, I'd love to do that," I gushed.

What an amazing moment of irony for me. Here I was, huge Uncle Nick, starting on a liquid diet, while my nephew was leaving a liquid diet and taking his first bite of solid food.

Afterward, my father and I said good-bye to our family, exchanged grasping hugs, and wiped away warm tears. I climbed into the van—

well, wedged my bulky torso between the seat and the steering wheel would be more like it—fired up the engine, and backed out of one life and drove off toward another one.

We headed north out of San Diego on Interstate 5, the main artery between America's Finest City—the home of *my* baseball team, the San Diego Padres—and the smoggy metropolis known as Los Angeles. My Padres were not playing the Dodgers that day—they were five hundred miles north, opening their season against the San Francisco Giants. I would be driving to the Bay Area after the Dodgers game to catch the Padres and the Giants on Wednesday evening.

At least I would be sitting in good seats at Dodger Stadium. Dr. Donald Miller, a pediatric physician and a comrade of mine, had a brother who was a Dodgers season-ticket holder, and his field-level seats were about ten rows off the third-base bag. Don was a huge baseball fan. He and I shared Padres season tickets, even though his allegiance switched to the Dodgers whenever the L.A. ball club rolled into town. I promised myself not to hold that against him for this game between the Dodgers and the Milwaukee Brewers.

Don was great to have on my team because he and I had spent several afternoons in December mapping out my cross-country baseball tour. What a logistical nightmare! My plan was to see more than one hundred games at thirty different major-league stadiums, and that involved some elaborate coordination. Some tickets had been mailed to me, and some were waiting at Will Call. Dad, who had been a semiprofessional soccer player in Greece, wasn't crazy about baseball (in fact, he would attend only a handful of games), so I lined up a friend or relative to join me at each game. It's no fun going to the ol' ballpark alone.

For the first game of my "Take a Swing at Weight Loss" tour, Dad made arrangements to visit with some Greek friends in L.A. while Don and I took in the game. My father took the helm of the USS *Spirit of Reduction* and dropped us off at Chavez Ravine, where we met Don's brother, Ross, who would give us a ride after the game.

"Where are our seats?" I asked Don as we made our way down Section 33 toward the third baseline.

"Row J," he replied.

I said a quick prayer. *Please let there be a seat on the aisle.* "Is there an aisle seat?" I asked.

"I don't think so."

Uh-oh. At Qualcomm Stadium in San Diego, our season seats included one on the aisle, which I sat in for obvious reasons.

My prayer went unanswered when I spotted three empty seats in the middle of the row. Don and Ross motioned for me to go first.

"Excuse me . . . excuse me . . . ," I said as the Dodgers fans leaned back and let me squeeze by. When I arrived at my seat, I was presented with a daunting task: squishing my broad backside into a hard plastic chair that measured twenty-one inches wide. Tough to do when you have a voluminous sixty-inch waist. As I dropped my rear end, I felt like I was stuffing an oversized pillow into a small cardboard box.

I knew what the guy next to me was thinking—*What a fatso!* I managed a weak smile. "I'm sorry to be crowding you," I mumbled.

Time to play baseball. I love the pageantry and optimism associated with Opening Day. Much like Easter, Opening Day is the ceremonial and symbolic end of winter and the start of spring, a time when every-one receives a fresh start and is 0–0 in the win-loss column.

Life is magnified on Opening Day. The sky is a deeper blue. The grass is a little greener. When the Marine Corps Color Guard marched in as the Dodgers and Brewers teams stood respectfully on the baselines, the excitement swirling among the 53,154 in attendance made me feel as though it were *my* Opening Day as well. I knew something wonderful would happen during the 2001 baseball season.

Batter up! I loved the sight of the first hitter—Milwaukee Brewers second baseman Ron Belliard—digging in, adjusting his batting glove, tapping his helmet, and stepping into the batter's box. Then I directed my attention to the Dodgers pitcher, Chan Ho Park, as he went through his own set of baseball rituals—sweeping the rubber with his right foot, touching the bill of his cap with his right hand, looking in for the sign, going into his windup, and hurling the horsehide. With the first pitch of the 2001 season, we were under way.

"Peanuts . . . git yer peanuts heeere!" screamed the teen vendor as he passed down our aisle. I tried to ignore the gawky kid hawking unshelled peanuts, but over the next two innings, wave after wave of food vendors passed by, pitching their junk-food wares: the popcorn guy, the Haagen-Dazs ice cream guy, the Cracker Jack guy, the Coke guy and . . . the Dodger Dog guy.

Dodger Dogs! I had forgotten about those, but anyone who had ever attended a ball game at Chavez Ravine knew about these footlong wieners. Suddenly, a wave of hunger assaulted me. I started getting light-headed again because I *really* wanted a Dodger Dog topped with mustard, ketchup, onions, and relish. The tangible benefits of the Last Supper had been cleansed from my intestinal tract that morning, which meant it was also Opening Day for the demons of hunger that were clenching and squeezing and grinding me. I think I saw a garland of Dodger Dogs spinning around my head.

Over the next few months, hundreds of people would ask me: "How can you travel around the country watching baseball games with all this food at the ballpark?" Great question. Baseball is probably the best sport to watch and eat simultaneously since there are long periods of inactivity between pitches. You're not sitting at the edge of your seat at the ballpark, which, I think, is one of the charms of the Grand Old Game. Eating helps pass the time, which is why we sing "Give me some peanuts and Cracker Jack, I don't care if I ever get back" during the seventh-inning stretch's "Take Me Out to the Ballgame." Despite all the eating that goes on at the ballpark, I still wanted to do a "Dr. Nick's Stadium Tour" because I loved the game so much. As for the food, I would have to do my best to ignore it, but that would happen anywhere I went.

In the third inning of a scoreless game, I put on my "Mr. Baseball Head" mask for the first time. The mask was a special gift from Stella Muller, one of my medical assistants. I thought it would be fun to wear the mask on the trip. "Mr. Baseball Head" certainly became a conversation starter, but it also attracted media attention like a moth is attracted to stadium lights. I slipped on the mask, which created a twitter in my section. Then I noticed several photographers in the camera pit next to the Dodgers dugout training their long Nikon lenses on me. There were also several Asian photographers, and then it dawned on me why: Chan Ho Park, a South Korean native, was pitching for the Dodgers, and the picture of an American wearing a whacked-out mask appealed to them. I waved and mugged for the cameras, but I wasn't about to stand up and show them my girth.

I turned my attention back to the game. Sure, I was longing for food, but that was offset by a sense of excitement. For the first time in years, I did not have a pager on my waist, did not have patients waiting to see me, did not have any staff meetings to attend, did not have any medical meetings to fly to, and did not have the daily piles of patient charts to plow through. In some ways, I felt like the happiest and luckiest man alive. The decision to combine doing something good for my health while doing something I totally enjoyed was feeling more and more like a brilliant idea to me.

The only cloud on the horizon was those vendors peddling their cotton candy and chocolate malts and Dodger Dogs. I fantasized about tackling one, tying him up with rope, and eating his stash of food. Then I remembered the photographers with their long lenses.

I snapped out of my daydream. We had a real pitchers' duel going—a scoreless tie through six innings. One of the game's story lines was how the fans would treat Dodgers left fielder Gary Sheffield. During spring training, Sheffield had drawn the wrath of the media and the fans for saying that since the Dodgers were unwilling to re-negotiate his contract (baseball talk for paying him more money), he might not "try" too hard when the game was on the line.

From the pregame introductions to each time Sheff came to the plate, boos cascaded down to him from the upper deck. We're talking Booville USA. The Dodgers fans didn't hold back their hostility—and this was one of their players!

Then, in the bottom of the sixth inning, Sheffield hit a monstrous home run over the centerfield fence, and you wouldn't believe how fast the boos turned to cheers. Fans were cheering, "Gar-ee, Gar-ee" as he rounded the bases. And that's how the game stood up—a 1–0 victory decided by a Gary Sheffield bomb.

As I watched the postgame celebration on the field, I thought I was witnessing Gary Sheffield's redemption day. I identified with him because I thought that one day *I* would experience redemption when

I lost—gulp—230 pounds. One day the funny looks and sneering comments that I heard as a fat person would turn to cheers, and I would receive pats on the back and "Attaboys" just like Gary Sheffield was receiving.

That evening, Dad and I drove toward the California coast and north on Highway 101. Doug Murphy, a med school buddy from my days at the University of California at San Diego (UCSD), had invited me to stay with him and his wife, Tamara, at their home in Cambria,

a central California coastal town. On the drive north, I felt upbeat about how the trip was unfolding.

My season to lose weight had begun.

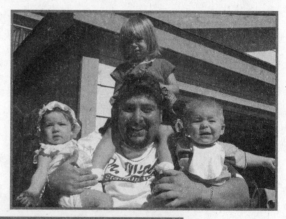

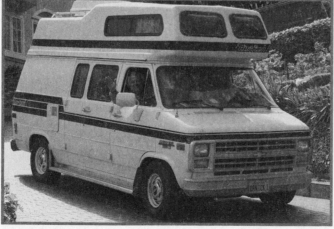

After saying good-bye to my nieces Nicole and Sophie and nephew Joey, Dad and I hopped into the USS *Spirit of Reduction* on a weight-loss journey that I didn't know how would end.

CHAPTER THREE

TRAVELING THROUGH BIG SUR COUNTRY

Monday, April 2
Cambria, California

I wasn't doing well when I veered the USS *Spirit of Reduction* into the Murphys' driveway. My body was transmitting weird signals after being deprived of food for the better part of two days.

When I stepped onto terra firma to greet Doug and Tamara, I felt as though I were having an out-of-body experience. My hands trembled slightly. My head spun like my office centrifuge. My gastric juices pumped like a piston, and my brain kept double-checking with my stomach as if to say, *Are you sure there's no food in there?*

I needed to get something into my digestive system. I had quaffed one protein shake that morning. That, along with a few whiffs of peanuts, popcorn, and Dodger Dogs at Chavez Ravine, wasn't doing it for me.

"Great to see you, Doug," I said as I gave him a bear hug after kissing Tamara on the cheek. You know how some guests ask to use the bathroom after they arrive? I needed a kitchen. "Hey Doug, you wouldn't mind if I used your blender, would you?" I asked. I held up a chocolate protein packet along with a diet chocolate soda and waved them at him.

"Sure, let's get you fixed up," Doug said graciously. I felt bad for cutting our greetings short, but I had the World's Ultimate Munchies growling in the pit of my stomach. Doug led me to the kitchen and lifted a blender from a kitchen cabinet. "Is there anything else you need?" he asked.

"Ice! I need ice. They make my shakes thicker when added to the blender."

"Sure." Doug opened the freezer, sensing the tone of urgency in my voice.

I had my protein shake whipped up in no time. "Umm, this hits the big empty spot," I said as Tamara led my father and me to the living room. "How's the trip going?" she asked.

"Great, just great," I said as I recounted the day's events. Thus started a special evening of hospitality. The Murphys were the first of more than 120 family members, college friends, medical school colleagues, ex-employees, baseball buddies, and friends of friends who would invite us into their homes to visit and/or spend the night with them over the next eight months.

When I began planning my weight-loss odyssey, I wanted to do more than watch baseball games, travel around the country, lose weight, and become healthier. I wanted to reconnect with friends and family. I had neglected some important relationships over the years, and I needed to right that wrong. In the Greek culture, visiting with loved ones and old acquaintances was something we called *koinonia*—the Greek word for fellowship. That's where the word kinship comes from, as Gus Portokalos from the movie My Big Fat Greek Wedding would say.

We certainly encountered *koinonia* with immediate family and complete strangers—people referred to us because they were friends of our friends. More than once I heard people say, "You're going through Ames, Iowa? Then you just have to stay with my old college roommate. He'd love to have you."

"No, really. We would be imposing," I would reply.

"Trust me, Freddie would love to meet you. I'm going to make the phone call right now."

That's what often happened, and over the upcoming months, I wouldn't believe how many people opened their homes and their hearts to us. On this particular evening in Cambria, Doug and Tamara Murphy happened to be the first to extend hospitality. After I finished downing my shake, Tamara placed a cup of tea with artificial sweetener in front of me for my "dessert."

Tamara sipped from a mug of lemon zinger tea. "Nick," she began, "I can't tell you how glad I am to see you here because I've been really worried about you. I've been praying for years that you would finally do something about your health and well-being."

"Years?" I asked, suddenly feeling humbled that someone would go to the trouble to actually pray about my sorry physical state.

Tamara nodded her head. "Yes, years, Nick. I think this idea you have about driving around the country watching baseball games while you go on this diet is wonderful. I hope that it works, too, because you're putting yourself on the line."

I didn't know what to say, although I must have straightened my shoulders a bit. I could feel an element of accountability creeping into my psyche, a feeling that I was responsible for what would happen during the next eight months. Everything was up to me. Would I give it a good start, only to begin eating again and fall back into my old habits? That's what had happened dozens of times before whenever I had started a diet. Or would I see this through and return to San Diego weighing hundreds of pounds less than I did now?

Frankly, I didn't know what would happen. The incident out in the Murphys' driveway with the shaky hands and light-headed queasiness didn't sit well with me. If that's how I felt after *two* days, what shape was I going to be in two weeks from now? Two months? Would I be a walking zombie, so whacked out by hunger that I couldn't put two sentences together? I couldn't imagine what would happen.

"What are your plans for tomorrow?" Doug asked.

"We're going to drive up Highway 1 to San Francisco. We have tickets to the Giants game against the Padres on Wednesday night."

"That worked out well," Doug said with a smile. He knew I was a big Padres fan.

I grinned. "It certainly did."

Tuesday, April 3
Somewhere Along Highway 1 in Central California

Highway 1 is a 122-mile-long ribbon of asphalt hugging the rugged cliffs of central California that plunge into power-mad surf. Flanked by dense pine forests to the east and glorious, sea-sculpted vistas to the west, I knew that our drive would give Dad and me a chance to reconnect with nature and California's most beautiful, unpopulated coastline.

We didn't drive long before making our first stop at Hearst Castle, just eight miles north of the Murphy home. Dad and I really wanted to take a tour of the magnificent 115-room mansion, where craftsmen and artisans had labored twenty-eight years, from the 1930s to the 1950s, to create a resplendent estate for William Randolph Hearst, the newspaper mogul. Unfortunately, the morning tours were sold out, so we wandered around the visitors center.

I enjoyed the exhibits displaying various aspects of the Hearst Castle. I was especially fascinated with the Refectory, or main dining hall inside the castle. Renaissance tapestries hung on the walls in a massive room fit for Henry VIII and his court. The captions explained that William Randolph Hearst loved to preside over lavish Saturday night dinners with forty of his closest friends, many of them Hollywood celebrities who had flown up the coast for the weekend. For a fleeting moment, I fantasized about being invited to one of Hearst's decadent affairs and joining him at the middle of the long table, regaling others with stories while I dug into a Ruth's Chris porterhouse steak for two.

Then I snapped out of it. I had to get out of there! Dad and I exited the visitors center and resumed our drive up Highway 1, which turned out to be everything that travel guidebooks promised it would be. We stopped numerous times at scenic lookouts to take pictures and soak in the breathtaking natural beauty before us. Big Sur country felt good on this windy spring day.

Dad and I took a detour and paid the $7.75 toll to tour the famed

17-Mile Drive through Pebble Beach, but we made good time because one of Dad's "friends"—the owner of a Greek restaurant in Monterrey called the Epsilon—was waiting for us. Our family joke was that Dad knew every Greek restaurant owner in California.

We drove up to the Epsilon and were welcomed like long-lost relatives. "You must come to our house," the owner said to us. "You just have to meet my mother, and we have some delicious Greek food waiting for you."

Great. Just what I wanted to hear. I started to protest, saying we really needed to get on the road, but Dad would have none of it. We couldn't turn our backs on *koinonia,* could we?

"We'd love to visit," I heard myself saying.

We stepped into their wonderful home just as plates of roasted lamb, broiled potatoes, rice, and a Greek salad were being set on a large table.

"Please, have something to eat," said the matriarch of the family.

"No, I can't," I replied. "I'm on a special diet."

"Come on, you have to eat something. Otherwise, you're going to die. How can you live without eating?"

"No, really, I'm on this serious diet, and I can't eat any food."

"You can't eat any food? What kind of diet is that? You have to eat something."

I knew she meant well, but she insisted that I accept her hospitality while I insisted that I couldn't eat anything. The thought that I could actually exist without eating solid food did not compute with my hosts. "Ah, Nick, you must eat. We eat to live, right?" said the matriarch.

"That's true, but I can't eat because I'm on this liquid diet, so the answer is no. What part of *oxi* [pronounced o-hee] do you not understand?" I said with a twinkle in my eye.

This declaration created an uproar. As only the Greeks can do, the discussion became quite animated for the next fifteen minutes as people talked with their hands and gestured that I *had* to eat because I would die if I didn't eat anything. I maintained my position until my hosts finally understood that I was serious—I could not eat and would not eat.

That didn't stop Dad, however, who filled a plate high with delicious food. He had no more than finished his last bite when I said we had to go. Again, in the Greek culture, this was rude behavior because we were expected to sit and visit for a while, but I had a radio interview with a San Diego talk-show host at 8 p.m., and we needed to be in Sebastopol (a good hour north of the Golden Gate Bridge), where we would be staying with the Foster family. This would be my first radio interview, and I was looking forward to chitchatting with the host for twenty-five minutes or so. The radio host, who said he had seen the same *North County Times* article as George Niece, called me prior to the Last Supper and said he would like to have me on the show several times during my weight-loss odyssey.

We arrived at the Foster home in Sebastopol—their son Willy and I had been best friends since med school—ten or fifteen minutes before my interview. I was a little nervous since I had never done live radio before, but the host put me at ease. In fact, I warmed up to the topic because I was talking about something I knew well—myself. I enjoyed the radio interview so much that during one station break, I wondered if my hunger for attention was greater than my hunger for food.

I was still aching from hunger and ready for bed after a long day on the road. Our hosts put Dad and me in Willy and his brother Wesley's old bedroom, equipped with two twin beds from when they were kids. I looked at the flimsy old twin bed as though it were covered with bedbugs. Why was that? I hadn't slept in one since high school. I was simply too big and too heavy for a twin bed.

I ever so gently eased my body onto the bed, worried that a quick movement would turn it into a splintered pile of toothpicks. All night long, I was careful to sleep on my side and not move, lest I crash through the bed boards and onto the floor. I slept poorly.

Compounding my discomfort was a recurring nightmare where I kept spilling off the edge of the twin bed, only to fall into a dark abyss of flavorless protein shakes.

Wednesday, April 4
San Francisco

I woke up not looking forward to the day because I planned to exercise—on purpose—for the first time since, oh, I had huffed and puffed my way around the track during PE classes at Tenafly High School in New Jersey. I avoided exercise the same way writers avoid clichés—like the plague.

I knew that if I was planning to lose 150, 200, or 250 pounds—it was so much weight that I didn't want to think about it—then drinking low-calorie protein shakes wasn't going to do it. I understood that the best and fastest way to lose weight was actually simple: Eat fewer calories, and exercise more. I was going in the right direction by decreasing the amount of calories I was taking in. I calculated that I had been eating around 5,600 calories a day prior to the Last Supper. How did I arrive at that figure? Since I weighed 467 pounds, my body needed approximately 12 calories per pound per day to maintain that weight. (I told you I ate a lot!) With the start of my diet regimen on April Fools' Day, twice-a-day protein shakes delivered just 800 calories.

Ergo, I stood a good chance to start losing weight right away since I had cut my caloric intake by nearly 5,000 calories a day. No wonder I was feeling so hungry!

But I couldn't depend on protein shakes to help me reach my weight-loss goal of 230 pounds. I needed to start exercising. I needed to stoke up a stone-cold furnace that hadn't been fired up in years. Exercise would be the one-two punch my body needed to start burning up reserves of fat.

But how do you exercise when you're on the road? Walking for an hour or two seemed undisciplined and haphazard. I couldn't pack a home gym into the USS *Spirit of Reduction*. Then, a month before my departure, Dick High, a Palomar Family YMCA board member in Escondido, heard about my upcoming trip. In recognition of my service as a community health physician and because he wanted to do something nice for me, he presented me with a one-year membership good at any YMCA in the country.

Perfect, I thought. Every town with more than two stoplights has a Y.

"When would you like the one-year membership to start?" asked Dick, perhaps thinking that I wanted to get a head start on my weight-loss odyssey by exercising before I left.

That was a foreign concept to me. I hadn't exercised in years. "How about Sunday, April 1?" I said.

Now I was mentally preparing myself for my first official workout. We drove into downtown San Francisco, where Dad dropped me off at the Central YMCA on Polk Street. He had made arrangements to meet another Greek "friend" who owned the Salonika, a Greek restaurant on the corner of Polk and California.

Meanwhile, I wandered into the Central Y feeling like Mommy

had dropped me off at kindergarten on the first day of class and left me to fend for myself. I presented my newly minted YMCA card and was directed to some lockers. I wasn't planning to change; my "Dr. Nick's Stadium Tour" T-shirt and XXXXXXL gym pants were all I had. Besides, shorts were not an option because shorts were designed for people with knees, not for pillars of hanging flesh with no curvature.

I stepped into the main exercise room—a fitness palace of stair-steppers, cross-trainers, treadmills, weight machines, and free weights. People were jogging at a rapid pace on the treadmills or bouncing up and down on the cross-trainers. At one end, racquetball players hustled after a blue ball. The exercise area was a beehive of activity because the noontime crowd had arrived.

I had never felt so self-conscious in my life. I sensed that every person was thinking, What's a gargantuan guy like that doing here? I wasn't feeling physically well, either. The blahs had definitely set in after three days without solid food. I wanted to take a nap, not exercise.

But I was here to get my heart rate up. I figured I would start with the simplest approach—walking on a treadmill. Anyone could do that, right? But I couldn't even remember the last time I'd stepped on a treadmill.

I spotted an empty one and approached it as if I knew what I was doing. I feared that a buff athletic trainer with washboard abs and muscles on top of his muscles would appear at any moment and ask whether I needed any help. I would have been mortified if that had happened. Thankfully, I was left alone.

How do you work the thing? I thought. *You could start by reading the directions.* I began pressing buttons on the computerized screen. For my weight, I tapped in 467, but the machine went *Tilt!*, notifying me that the maximum weight capacity was 350. Another indignity, but I brushed it off. I touch-typed 350, while saying—with some glee—to the treadmill, Guess what? You're going to enjoy the weight of an extra 117 pounds. Next I punched in the time: thirty minutes. For speed, I pressed the button for 1.5 mph—pretty slow, but not the slowest setting. One mph was the slowest.

After pressing the last button, the treadmill roared to life. I managed to step on and stay on my feet. A speed of 1.5 mph seemed leisurely—for about fifteen seconds. Then I started huffing and puffing as much as the guy on the treadmill next to me—which, I noticed, was set on 6 mph! I held the railing for support as I struggled to keep putting one foot in front of the other. In no time, sweat poured off my forehead and ran in rivulets down my face, which had turned beet red. I concentrated on putting one foot in front of the other and keeping up with the moving walkway.

I was never so thankful to see thirty minutes pass. I stepped off the treadmill and took inventory as I gulped large breaths of air. My knees hurt. My ankles ached. And my ego was shattered.

For the better part of fifteen years, the most physical activity I had done was lifting a fork to my mouth or pushing back from a dinner table. I didn't mind patrolling mall parking lots for an extra five minutes if that would land me a parking space closer to the front door. Doing physical exercise was not on my radar screen. If I burned any calories at all, that happened passively, not from physical activity. I smiled, though I was in complete misery. I had done it. I had exercised for the first time since high school, and I felt the same euphoric sense of accomplishment that Rocky did when he bounded up the steps of the Philadelphia Museum of Art.

Getting stronger . . .

GETTING THE GOOD SEATS

Dad and I arrived at Pacific Bell Park three hours before game time, which would become our custom whenever we visited a new baseball stadium. We didn't want to be rushed. The first thing I did was walk around the perimeter of the ballpark while Dad rested his sore knees in the RV. Pac Bell had several unusual features. The Coca-Cola Fan Lot (I know, all these corporate sponsorships) had tons of great stuff for kids: superslides, a mini-Pac Bell Park where kids could take batting practice against pitching machines throwing softballs, and a place to test how fast they could throw the ball. A raised mezzanine ringed much of the outfield area, including right field, which overlooked McCovey's Cove, where many a Barry Bonds home run landed only to be fished out by Portuguese water dogs. Two other aspects intrigued me—an inspirational nine-foot statue of America's greatest living ballplayer, Willie Mays, in front of Pac Bell and a twenty-six-foot-high, thirty-two-foot-wide replica of an old-time four-fingered, baseball glove beyond the left-center alley.

After walking the perimeter, I met up with Dad at the Will Call window, where two tickets were supposed to be left in my name. I held my breath because (1) I couldn't be sure if the tickets would be there, and (2) I had no idea where our seats would be.

During the off-season, I had been invited to a special reception for Padres season ticket holders at Qualcomm Stadium. There were several Padres front office people in attendance, including team president Larry Lucchino.

It was one of those stand-up affairs where people mill around nibbling hors d'oeuvres and nursing drinks until several speeches and presentations are made. Good PR for the Padres, who needed it because they had inhabited the National League West cellar the previous season.

I bumped into Lee Hofacre, whom I knew from the Palomar Pomerado Health Foundation, which raised money for our local hospital system. I made a beeline over to Lee and initiated small talk with him.

Naturally, he asked me what I was up to, and I casually mentioned that beginning April 1, I was planning to not eat solid food for eight months while I traveled around the country watching baseball games. Lee's eyes lit up.

"Larry's got to hear this," he said, and before I knew it, I was being introduced to Larry Lucchino of the Padres.

"Larry, you've got to meet the ultimate baseball fan, and you won't believe what he's going to do this upcoming season," said Lee. "Dr. Nick here is going to visit all thirty major-league baseball stadiums while he goes on this diet."

That introduction piqued Larry's interest, and for the next five or ten minutes, he listened and smiled while I outlined my "Take a Swing at Weight Loss" tour. He seemed genuinely interested.

"Listen," he said when I was done, "if there is anything I can do to help out, please let me know."

Actually, Larry, there is something you can do . . . As a baseball fan, I knew that there were certain stadiums—Baltimore's Camden Yards, Cleveland's Jacobs Field, San Francisco's Pac Bell Park, and Chicago's Wrigley Field—that were tough tickets. They were often sold out before the season started, and even if tickets were available, they were what fans call "Bob Uecker" seats—three decks high and deep in the right-field corner.

"Thanks for your offer, Mr. Lucchino," I began. "Actually, if somebody in the front office could help me coordinate getting some tickets, that would be great. I'm not asking to receive them free, but if there is any way you could help me buy some tickets, that would be great."

"Absolutely," he said. "Let me introduce you to someone who can help you out," said the Padres team president.

I was introduced to Kurt Varricchio, a young and earnest group sales representative. His ears didn't perk up when I began telling him my story, however. He probably felt that he had to listen to this inflated monstrosity of a human being telling him about his grandiose plan to drive around the country watching baseball games while he went on a diet. *Yeah right, and the pope's Jewish. Let me know when you come down off that stuff you're smoking.*

I have to credit Kurt. Although he might have been thinking that I was off my rocker, he had been asked by his boss to help me out. "Here's my card," he said. "I need you to send me an e-mail with each date and each stadium on your itinerary. Once I get that, I'll look into getting those tickets for you."

Now, Pac Bell Park was the first time I was relying on tickets organized by Kurt—seats that I had paid for. Would the tickets be waiting for me? Where would I be sitting?

Bingo! A pair of ducats waiting in my name. Dad and I walked through the turnstile, and holy moley, our seats were field-level beauties—seven rows behind the Padres dugout, in an area usually reserved for VIPs, scouts, players' wives and friends, and league officials. In other words, tickets not available to the general public.

There were still another two hours before game time, so Dad and I started another custom—walking around the interior of the ballpark, soaking up the atmosphere, and looking at every nook and cranny of Pacific Bell, which opened in the year 2000. When we returned to our seats, the players were starting to limber up and take batting practice. These were the best seats I'd ever had at a major-league game. I walked up to the railing separating the stands and the players. It seemed as if I could reach out and touch Tony Gwynn as he stepped out of the dugout to begin his pregame warm-up.

But I didn't ask for autographs, nor would I bother other players with autograph requests during the trip. Instead, I took plenty of pictures with my digital camera. I also sought out an usher, because I wanted Dad to take a picture of an usher and me at every ballpark we visited. Why ushers? Because they were always agreeable to having their picture taken with me. I also figured that each usher-and-Nick photo would provide a photographic sequence of how much weight I was losing. (See the appendix for all thirty photos of me with the ushers.)

I loved the view from such great seats, although hunger pains were grinding me. It didn't help matters that our hoity-toity section had well-dressed waiters and waitresses—no high-school kids peddling their peanuts—who took orders from ticket holders and then returned with some of the most mouthwatering food I had seen in a long time. I'm talking sushi, gourmet burgers, garlic fries, and—a San Francisco treat—clam chowder in a sourdough bread bowl.

I made my first JumboTron appearance at Pac Bell. Like most ballparks with JumboTron screens, TV cameras sweep the stands between innings showing Joe Fan and his family eating cotton candy or a couple dancing to the music. Between innings one time, I stood up with my "Mr. Baseball Mask" and was delighted to see myself on the JumboTron. Besides serving as a magnet for TV and stadium cameras, the mask provided a prophylactic guard over my mouth, lest the temptation to inhale some food became too much to handle.

Alas, my Padres took one on the chin in a bizarre finish. With the score 7–7 in the bottom of the ninth inning, Giants pinch runner Calvin Murray stood on second base when Shawon Dunston blooped a single to center field. Murray's feet pedaled so hard that he crashed into the infield dirt before he reached third base, but he quickly sprang up and began rounding third for home as the Giants third-base coach waved him on. Murray slipped a second time, however, this time on the dewy grass, and had to scramble back to third base. Padres catcher Ben Davis, who had gloved the relay throw, fired the ball to third base, trying to nail the diving base runner.

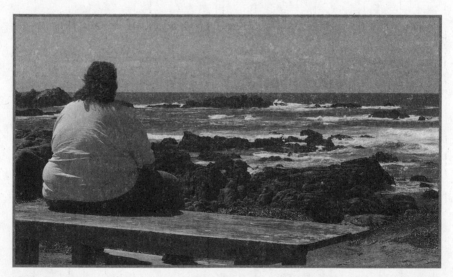

As hunger pains assaulted me those first few days, I contemplated my future along the Central California coast.

Unfortunately, third baseman Phil Nevin couldn't glove the throw, and the ball skittered twenty feet up the left-field baseline. Murray jumped to his feet and just beat the throw home.

The next day, the newspapers quoted Giants pitcher Shawn Estes as saying that Calvin Murray looked like a "pig on ice" when he slipped and fell twice trying to score the winning run.

A pig on ice.

Just what I needed to inspire me. Another fat joke.

CHAPTER FOUR

THE
BLACK HOLE

D ad and I left San Francisco and drove to a quaint Napa
Valley town called Healdsburg, where we were invited to
stay with another buddy from my med school days, Dr.
Steven Vargas.

Steve, I had to admit, had done pretty well for himself. He lived on a
Tuscany-like estate tucked away in ten rolling acres of vineyards, lined
with grapes destined for California's wine market. Dad and I were shown
our guest rooms, and when I turned in for the night, I heard several wild
turkeys making a nuisance in the courtyard. The *gobble-gobbles*
prompted a dream in which I fantasized about shooting those turkeys

and celebrating Thanksgiving a little early this year. "What's wrong with having Thanksgiving on April 6?" I wrote in my journal the following morning.

At lunchtime, our host invited us to a snooty French restaurant in Healdsburg where the smaller the entrée, the higher the price. Eating at a restaurant like that would have bummed me out in my bad old days, when *quantity* was more important than quality, but I shrugged it off since I was ordering only something to drink.

After giving the matter some thought—this would be my meal that afternoon—I settled on diet lemon tea. Man, that drink tasted great, but with each tiny sip, I fantasized that I was drinking liquid turkey. The lack of solid food was getting to me. I was five days into my all-liquid diet, and my body was protesting loud and clear: *I want food! I want food!* I must have been feeling the same withdrawal pains that strung-out druggies face when trying to kick heroin or crack cocaine. Waves of hunger pains assaulted my body, and a headache pounded my temples with a steady drumbeat. As a practicing physician, I knew what to expect, but boy, it was something actually experiencing it.

Fortunately, I had a game to attend that night, which gave me something to look forward to. It was Opening Day for the Oakland A's at Network Associates Coliseum—the dual-purpose stadium that was also home to the football team I hated most, the Oakland Raiders. Every San Diego Chargers fan knows about the infamous "Black Hole," the home of the Silver and Black.

When I arrived at Oakland stadium, my mood was as black as a Raiders jersey. My hunger wasn't hunger any longer—it was a searing physical pain, like I had a black hole in my stomach. For tonight's game, I invited Dr. Cheryl Ho to join me. I had mentored Cheryl when

I was a voluntary faculty member at the UCSD School of Medicine. Now she was doing her internship at a nearby hospital in Oakland.

An usher escorted us to our seats in the club section overlooking home plate. "Here are your seats," he said. "The dinner buffet is open until the fifth inning."

Did he say what I thought he said?

"What dinner buffet?" I asked.

"All club ticket holders receive a dinner buffet. It's part of your ticket."

Letting a free meal pass by didn't sit well with me. Our family had come from humble economic means, so saying no to free food was like dropping your wallet and not bending over to pick it up.

"Where's the buffet?" I inquired, as if knowing where the buffet line was would make me feel better, but it didn't. I still hurt.

"Through the doors back there," the usher replied, jerking his thumb.

"Thank you," I mumbled.

Cheryl, to her credit, was sensitive to my plight. "Nick, I don't have to have the dinner buffet."

"No, go ahead," I said, touched at her sensitivity.

"You won't mind if I eat in front of you?"

"Absolutely not, Cheryl. Go for it. I'll be okay."

When she came back to her seat, she held a white Styrofoam plate with a modest assortment of sliced turkey, potato salad, green salad, and a dessert cookie. That would have been an appetizer for me one week ago, but now it looked like nature's bounty.

"Can I smell your food?" I asked good-naturedly, but inside, I was dying.

When she nodded yes, I leaned over and inhaled the aroma. I pretended to get the vapors, which made her laugh, but then the hunger pains returned with a vengeance. My mood dipped even further, and with the arrival of light rain, I bundled up against the damp cold. Cool April evenings in the Bay Area could be quite depressing, I judged.

"Last call for the buffet line," the usher announced at the end of the fourth inning. The more I thought about it, the more I could not let go of the free food. I knew Dad would appreciate a plate, so I excused myself to make a pass through the buffet line. I piled one plate high with sliced chicken, sausage, different cheeses and breads, various salads, and several cookies. Then I took another Styrofoam plate and covered it. As much as I was tempted to snitch a bite, though, I remained strong. I knew Dad would appreciate the thoughtful gesture after the game. It was free food, after all.

A steady rain pelted us for the next few innings. Cheryl excused herself in the seventh inning, saying she had to work early in the morning. I told her good-bye. "I'd leave with you," I said, "but I told Dad I would meet him twenty minutes after the game."

"No problem," Cheryl said.

After the final out, I walked out of the Oakland stadium wearing my backpack and cradling Dad's dinner with two hands. The light rain had turned into a downpour, and I hustled to find the USS *Spirit of Reduction* at our rendezvous point—the BART stop. I was getting soaked since I didn't have an umbrella. I spotted Dad and waved. As I approached the van, I walked around the rear so I could hand him his meal through the driver-side window, but then disaster struck. I slipped on a backed-up drainage gate and took a pratfall. Dad's plate of food leaped out of my hands and smashed into the back of the van, while I fell into a huge puddle. Lying on my back, soaked to the bone, I was stunned by the rapid turn of events. I felt horrible that Dad's dinner was ruined and ticked that I was wet and cold, lying in a river of water. To add insult to injury, Dad started up the engine, and a belch of exhaust blew into my face.

It can't get any worse than this, I thought. I hated being cold, I hated being wet, and I hated being hungry. Life stank, and I felt sorry for myself. Tears rolled down my cheeks, and I couldn't find the desire to get up. I was no better than an alcoholic lying drunk in the gutter. I had reached rock bottom. I would never lose any weight.

I pulled myself up and yanked open the passenger door. Dad started laughing when he saw me, dripping water from head to toe. "Nick, you look like a wet dog—"

"Dad, it's not funny," I choked, trying not to cry in front of him.

"What's wrong, son?"

"Dad, I . . . I fell." I wiped my eyes with the back of my hands. It was embarrassing to cry in front of my father, but I couldn't help myself. "I brought you a plate of food for dinner, but now it's ruined."

"That's okay," my father soothed. "You'll be okay."

I stepped into the rear of the USS *Spirit of Reduction* and changed into a dry "Dr. Nick's Stadium Tour" T-shirt and gray sweatpants. Then we stopped by a mini-mart, where I purchased a diet soda in a thirty-two-ounce cup of ice. I quickly gulped the soft drink and used the ice to make my second protein shake of the day.

Each swig delivered much-needed relief. I leaned back and felt blood rush back into my head. *Ah, this feels good.* Then another thought—an empowering one—came to my mind: If you can survive this, you can survive anything. Bring it on.

DREAM ON

Dad drove us to the Greek Assembly of God Church in Oakland, where we would camp that night in the parking lot. The cheap place to stay was borne out of another of Dad's Greek connections.

A steady rain pelted the van, and I fell asleep thinking about the buffet line back at the Oakland ballpark. I dreamed about walking past the impressive display of food, piling my plate high with drumsticks and chicken breasts, antipasto salad, fettuccini with Italian sausage, breads, salads—anything I could lay my hands on. I sampled food along the way because I was so hungry. Then I woke up, sure that I had eaten. My dream was that vivid.

I fell back asleep and entered another dream. This time, I checked into a five-star luxury hotel, where I was happily ensconced in a penthouse suite. I called room service and ordered a king's banquet to be delivered to my room, but when the knock came, I couldn't open the door! The knocking grew louder and louder, and I could hear the valet saying, "Room service! Room service!" Still, I could not open the door. Delicious food was so close but yet so far.

I woke up in a panicked state, and then I heard banging on the side of the van. "Open up! Oakland police!"

I was sleeping on a pull-out bed in the rear of the van, and when I parted the curtains, the brightest light flashed in my eyes. "Open up immediately!" barked a police officer.

I unlocked the side door.

"It's against the law to camp out in city limits," the policeman announced.

"But we have permission from the church to park our van here," I replied.

"Yes, I called and got permission," Dad chimed in, adding he was supposed to tune the church piano in the morning. When the cop heard Dad's accented English, he figured the story was on the up-and-up. "Okay, I guess you can stay," he said.

Dad tuned the church piano in the morning and joined me for the afternoon game between the A's and the Anaheim Angels. This would be the first of only a handful of games that we would attend together during the 2001 season. Although he didn't accompany me on every leg of the trip, he did the baseball tour to support me, which was a selfless act.

We had club seats again, which included a lunch buffet. I was feeling a little better, and watching Dad eat a good meal lifted my spirits. He hadn't slept well, what with all the commotion from the local cops, so when he asked in the fourth inning if he could leave and take a nap in the van, I told him that was a good idea.

When he left, it dawned on me that the buffet line was open for another inning. For the next twenty minutes, my gastric juices flowed like the Mississippi River at flood stage. I was in the ballpark all alone, and behind me a gorgeous buffet was beckoning me . . . tempting me . . . luring me. Beads of sweat formed on my forehead. This was where the real challenge of obesity lay—the constant temptation. The constant pressure to say no wore on my nerves.

That afternoon, all sorts of bad thoughts entered my consciousness. I told myself that I could easily sneak some food. Who would find out? Maybe a salad wouldn't be so bad. What was wrong with eating a few carrots dipped in ranch dressing? I played with each food-related thought, dissecting it like a physician studying a tissue sample. I lined up several rationalizations regarding the propriety of eating a "little something": No one would be the wiser, it wouldn't hurt me in the long run; and some solid food would boost my sagging spirits. This was a slippery slope. Had I made a compromise here, I could easily have slid back into my old habits. One little exception could have easily led to a monumental "relapse."

I didn't know it at the time, but this was a real hinge moment for me. As I wavered, I was torn between the desire of my flesh—to eat—and the desire of my spirit—to remain true to my liquid fast. I now believe that I didn't fall to temptation that afternoon for two reasons: the countless prayers of family, friends, and even strangers who had read the newspaper stories or seen the TV news features on my baseball tour, and the accountability of my hometown community of Escondido.

Several community groups, including my own health clinic, had honored me with a dinner and a celebrity roast one week prior to my weight-loss trip. Three hundred people showed up for the gala affair, and proceeds from the event were earmarked for health and arts programs to benefit disadvantaged children in our community. Those in attendance were also given the opportunity to pledge $1 (or any amount they wanted) for every pound I lost to benefit the Escondido Community Health Center or the California Center for the Arts. When I remembered how people back home were counting on me to lose some serious weight, my resolve not to eat doubled.

I got up out of my seat and walked to . . . the bathrooms. I held my game ticket in my hand, and I thought for a long moment about flushing it down the toilet so I would no longer be tempted to graze at the buffet. But I was planning to have a scrapbook of all my game tickets, so I kept the ticket and walked out of the bathroom. I was resolute in my determination not to eat solid food, and I didn't, although hunger continued to gnaw at my stomach.

Sunday, April 8
Oakland, California

Dad and I attended services at the Greek Assembly of God Church, but I had a date that afternoon at another cathedral—this one dedicated to baseball. Dad opted not to go at the last moment, saying he would meet me after the game. I sold my extra ticket to some fellow in the parking lot. I gave him a good deal—$20 for a $25 ticket.

At least a buffet table wouldn't tempt me. I had a regular seat, though, and that was *not* the same as a club seat. Club seats were a few inches wider in Oakland; regular stadium seats had a standard width of nineteen inches. I didn't feel like squishing my rear end or pinching my thighs on metal armrests all afternoon. I thought about finding a seat in the club section, but then I noticed a handicapped area behind the field-level seats. I was handicapped, wasn't I? Maybe I didn't have a wheelchair, but I had a caboose that handicapped me from sitting in regular seats.

The handicapped section was lightly populated, but I noticed something interesting—several empty metal chairs without armrests. The folding chairs were apparently set there for the able-bodied folks assisting those in their wheelchairs.

"Mind if I sit here?" I asked one fellow in his wheelchair. He looked to have cerebral palsy.

"No, be . . . be my . . . my guest," he stuttered.

I sat down with a gloomy sense of despondency, feeling sorry for myself.

"Wha—what's your name?" the fellow asked.

"Nick. What's yours?"

"Paul. You . . . you like baseball?"

And we were off and running. We talked baseball for the next few innings, and the dark cloud hovering over me lifted. *Did I really have it so bad?* Paul, I realized, couldn't change his handicap, but I could.

"Can I get you something to eat?" I asked. "My treat."

"No, you . . . you don't—"

"Really, I insist. What would you like?"

That afternoon, I bought Paul a hot dog, a couple of sodas, a pretzel, and an ice-cream bar—whatever he wanted. Ballpark prices being what they are, that was a chunk of change, but I wanted to do something nice for the guy. He was providing me with companionship and a place to sit comfortably—two priceless commodities to me at that moment. In a sense, he ministered to me when I needed a lift. By the end of the game, we were good buddies who exchanged e-mail addresses.

LONG RIDE HOME

After the game, the plan called for us to drive back to San Diego, where I would catch the Padres' Opening Day game (my third in a week) Tuesday night at Qualcomm Stadium.

Driving through the flat and boring San Joaquin Valley late at night—during a pelting rainstorm—prompted an intense conversation between my father and me. It was all about food and my weight. Things had been building up for years, and I needed to get some things off my chest.

Dad was from the Old Country, a very strict, disciplinary guy, while my mom was always gracious and accepting. My father was never abusive to me, the oldest son, but I was a rascal as a kid, constantly testing the limits. Naturally, I was frequently and decisively disciplined whenever I stepped over the line.

My parents used food as a means to reward or discipline me. If I brought home a good report card, we would celebrate by going out to KFC and eating the biggest bucket of chicken you could buy. If I beat up my younger brothers, I was banished to my room without dinner. If I finished my homework to my father's satisfaction, I could get myself a treat, like cookies or ice cream. If I didn't listen to Mom, I got no dessert.

We experienced economic poverty and hardships growing up, but whenever something good happened, we celebrated the Greek way— with our mouths and our stomachs. When we had the money, we stacked the dinner table with mousaka (a beef, pasta, and eggplant casserole) or roasted lamb and broiled garlic potatoes. We would eat like it was Thanksgiving.

"I wish you hadn't raised me that way; I wouldn't be who I am," I said, my voice nearly cracking. "Look at me. I'm a fat tub of lard, and now I'm miserable. I'm hungry, I don't have any energy, and I don't think I'm losing any weight. Based on what I've gone through, so help me God, if I have lost five pounds or less . . ."

"Nick, don't say that," my father said quietly.

"No, I mean it, Dad. When I weigh myself tomorrow, if I have lost five pounds or less, then I'm going to a buffet as soon as I step off the scale. This is ridiculous. You can forget about this stupid diet."

Dad was shocked and saddened to hear the vehemence in my voice, but I was sick and tired of my fat body, sick and tired of the liquid diet I had been on for one week, and sick and tired of the emotional frustration I was feeling. I was angry about the deprivation I was going through, and I was sure I had lost absolutely no weight in the previous week. For all I knew, I could have gained a few pounds.

As we pulled into our driveway at 2:30 in the morning, I shuffled to my room and got ready for bed. The weigh-in later that morning would determine whether this had been a one-week experiment that ended in failure or the start of a long, difficult journey. In gambler's terms, I pushed all my chips into the center of the table. The weigh-in would determine everything.

Monday morning was Judgment Day.

Monday, April 9
Escondido, California

After a little more than three hours of sleep, I woke up suddenly at 6:30 a.m. with the same anxiety I felt whenever I had a major exam in med school. Actually, this felt more important. I felt that this was a test I had to pass to go on with my life. Everything was on the line.

I knew what was waiting for me in the bathroom: a pair of identical white medical-quality scales on which I had weighed myself eight days earlier and learned—to my horror—that I weighed 467 pounds. I rolled my mounds of flesh out of bed and lumbered to the bathroom, holding my breath. I voided so I could weigh as little as possible, and then I stepped out of my underwear. I looked at the two scales and whispered a prayer. I lifted my right foot and stepped on one scale, which shot toward the 350-pound mark until I slowly lifted my left foot off the ground and placed it on the other scale.

I closed my eyes and took a deep breath. I couldn't bear to look.

When I finally peeked, my body was trembling so badly that the numbers were swinging back and forth. I couldn't steady myself long enough to get a reading. At first, one scale said 300 and the other 150. My mind couldn't compute that simple math. Then I balanced myself, and the scales eventually evened out. Each read 225 pounds.

I had lost the ability to count. I couldn't figure out what 225 plus 225 was. *Wait a minute—that's 450 pounds!* My heart started racing. Did I lose seventeen pounds in one week? I had never heard of a human being losing seventeen pounds in one week, unless they had a tumor or lost a limb. I played with the scale, putting more weight on one leg versus the other, but every combination added up to 450 pounds.

Hee-haw! I lost seventeen pounds! I stepped off the scales and danced a little jig around the bathroom—just like if my Padres came from behind to win the game in the bottom of the ninth inning.

The commotion woke my parents and prompted them to investigate the hullabaloo. I quickly found some clothes and stepped out of the bathroom. "Mom, Dad, it's working. I lost seventeen pounds!"

They hugged me, and for the rest of the day, I was on cloud nine, calling my friends and telling the good news. I had aced the first of many pop quizzes.

Tuesday, April 10
Opening Day for the San Diego Padres

I began the day by inviting Margaret Georges, a seventy-something nurse who had just retired after devoting years to our community health clinic, out to breakfast at a local coffee shop. I deeply appreciated what this caring woman had selflessly done for my patients.

I now felt much more comfortable being around food, the odor of food, and the sight of food. Margaret, bless her heart, ordered a complete breakfast: scrambled eggs, country potatoes, muffin, and coffee, while I sat there with an iced tea and a glass of water with lemon.

That morning, I committed a new sin that I created myself—the sin of foodography. I defined *foodography* as "deriving great pleasure from watching other people eat." For the next eight months, I would commit the sin of foodography nearly every day.

My Padres opened their home season against the San Francisco Giants, but after Barry Bonds blasted a home run in the first inning, the Padres were handily defeated. I didn't care. I had won my game by seventeen pounds.

After the final out, I drove to the Escondido Community Health Center, from where I was taking a leave of absence, to witness a symbolic moment. My brother Phil was taking over my practice, and Dr. Jim Schultz would be handling my administrative duties. We took a picture of me passing the baton—in this case, a computer keyboard—to Phil and Jim. In many ways, this felt like a release point from my work commitments and would allow me to concentrate on my weight-loss tour.

The rest of the week, I attended every game of the Padres' six-game home stand and exercised at the Palomar Family YMCA, walking thirty minutes a day on a treadmill. The contraption no longer felt like something from outer space. Although I was still walking at a 1.5 mph pace, my body was slowly getting used to more exercise. What once had been an absolutely intolerable event was now at least bearable.

On Thursday afternoon, I invited Brad Wiscons to the house to meet with my entire family. I didn't know Brad very well, but he was a local activist involved in a variety of social initiatives benefiting those in our community who needed it the most. Brad had done what I was doing—drinking protein shakes and not eating any solid food. In the last six months, he had lost 133 pounds, dropping from 333 pounds to 200 pounds.

I invited Brad over to undergo an Yphantides family interrogation. Dad, Mom, several brothers, and my sister wanted to know if the protein shake diet really worked and what were the pros and cons. With our hectic schedules, this was our first chance to get together.

My family didn't stand on ceremony. "Brad, what effect did this diet have on your ability to have a bowel movement?" one of my brothers—who shall go nameless—asked.

Brad was nonplussed. "There were times supplementary fiber was necessary, and I can assure you that drinking plenty of water was of vital importance. Besides that, everything worked fine."

Another brother boldly asked Brad to lift up his shirt and show us his loose skin.

"I'll do you one better," Brad replied. He stood up and not only lifted his shirt, but he unbuckled his pants and allowed us to view his lower abdomen. His skin appeared loose and redundant as it contoured his body.

"Were you hungry?" my mother asked.

"Initially, I was famished. But as my body adjusted to the diet, it was surprisingly tolerable."

Yeah, yeah, whatever, I thought. Compared to me, Brad had been a scrawny 333-pounder, but I appreciated his honesty. My family needed to hear from Brad because they were a bit concerned for me. A year earlier, when I had brought up my idea of taking a year off from work and traveling around the country drinking protein shakes, they looked at me as though I should be locked up in the psychiatric ward at Palomar Medical Center. My family were not the only ones who thought I was whacked out. Almost universally I would receive the following response: You're going on a diet while going on a road trip and watching baseball games? Are you out of your mind? No offense, Nick, but that's the craziest thing I've ever heard. You've really gone off the deep end.

I replied that I knew my plan sounded crazy, but I needed to shake things up. I had decided that if I was going to change my weight, I had to change my life.

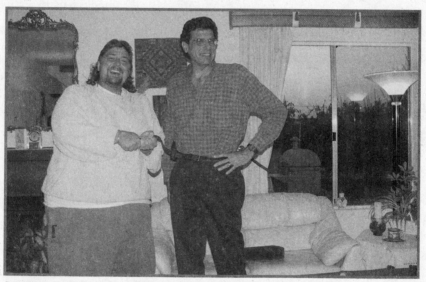

Brad Wiscons and I lost a collective 400 pounds that we hope to never find again.

Brad took me aside after the interrogation session was over. "I have no doubt that you're going to do this," he said. "Trust me. If I can do this, you can, too."

That encouraged me, and when I fired up the USS *Spirit of Reduction* for the next leg of my weight-loss odyssey, I was ready to see this thing through.

CHAPTER FIVE

REELING IN THE YEARS

Saturday, May 26
Newton, Massachusetts

Six weeks had passed since I left San Diego, and now I found myself in the Northeast for a happy family occasion. My brother Paul was marrying a lovely Greek girl named Eleni.

Paul, the second born and eighteen months younger than me, lived at the family home in Escondido and worked in sales management for a power electronics manufacturing firm headquartered in the Boston area. During a business trip to the home office in April 2000, he met Eleni while attending a service at the Greek Evangelical Church.

It was love at first sight. Call us traditional, but we have this thing in the Yphantides family: Marriage is once and for all, and the engagement is a critical part of the commitment process. How Paul asked Eleni to marry him is a doozy of a story.

Six months into their bicoastal courtship, Eleni flew out to San Diego. One afternoon they visited the Wild Animal Park, which is not far from our Escondido home. The Wild Animal Park, affiliated with the San Diego Zoo, has various shows during the day, including one involving an Australian galah, a pink-breasted cockatoo, named Yo-Yo.

Paul and Eleni settled into the Benbough Amphitheater with several hundred other people. They heard the trainer ask if anyone was willing to hold a dollar bill up and allow Yo-Yo to take it away—and return with it later.

More than a dozen raised their hands.

"Anyone willing to part with a five-dollar bill?" the trainer asked.

"I will," one fellow cried out.

"How about a twenty-dollar bill?" the trainer asked.

"Over here!" Paul yelled, while pointing at Eleni.

Eleni was very reluctant to stand up in front of hundreds of strangers since she was not one for the spotlight. She eagerly tried to pass the twenty-dollar bill back into Paul's hands, hoping that he would do it himself. With much fuss—and some vocal urging from the audience—Paul cajoled Eleni into standing up and stretching her right arm high in the air. A folded-up Andrew Jackson rested in the palm of her hand.

"Are you ready?" the trainer asked.

Eleni timidly nodded.

The trainer released the bird, which swooped into the air and dive-bombed toward Eleni. The Australian galah clasped its talons on the twenty-dollar bill and swooshed gracefully in a big arc before landing on the trainer's right arm.

The audience clapped in appreciation, but during the hubbub, the trainer switched the twenty-dollar bill with a one-dollar bill my brother had given him before the show.

"Now, let's see if the young lady receives back her money," the trainer said. With a dramatic lift of his arm, he beckoned Yo-Yo to start its return flight.

When the cockatoo dropped the greenback into Eleni's outstretched palm, the crowd applauded again. Eleni sat down in a hurry, thankful the ordeal was over. The trainer walked closer to Eleni. "Was your money returned to you?" he asked.

Eleni looked down at the unfolded paper bill.

"I'm . . . I'm not sure," she said, tension rising in her voice. "It's a dollar bill, but there's something written on it."

"What does it say?" the trainer inquired.

Eleni looked down. By now, her hands were trembling. "It says, 'This is the day that the Lord has made. Eleni, will you marry me?' "

The crowd melted, and I, along with fifteen other family members, jumped out of the bushes we had been hiding in—just in time to see Eleni hyperventilate. "Oh, my God, oh, my God," she cried, as she wrapped her arms around Paul's neck. My brother then bent to one knee and gazed into her eyes. "Will you marry me, Eleni?"

Yup, that's how we like to do marriage proposals in the Yphantides family. The poor girl was toxic with surprise and excitement.

Now we were on the other side of the country in Newton, Massachusetts, twenty miles east of Beantown, getting ready for the Big Day. I was so happy that I thought I was getting married. For the first time in my life, I didn't dread being part of a wedding. Why? Because I fit into a tuxedo. Not only that, a seamstress had to take in my rented tux to make it fit just so. Another reason for my giddiness was that I had lost seventy-five pounds and dipped under the four-hundred-pound barrier for the first time in what—fifteen years? I was feeling really good, like I was ready for the cover of GQ. I also felt good because I had worked out that morning at a local gym, walking on a treadmill for forty-five minutes at three miles per hour—double the rate I had started at in San Francisco.

Paul asked me to be the best man for the wedding and the master of ceremonies for the reception. They were married at the Greek Evangelical Church in one of Massachusetts' oldest church buildings before 350 family members and close friends. The wedding ceremony was officiated by the Greek Evangelical pastor, who pronounced the vows in Greek, followed by the English translation.

The reception was held at a nearby country club, complete with an elegant sit-down dinner and the usual frivolities of a Greek wedding experience. I was so dialed in to my diet that I found it easy not to eat, although my knees weakened when I saw the New England clam chowder and crab cakes served as a starter. I'm afraid I committed the sin of foodography, Northeastern style.

Looking back, I can honestly state that my brother's wedding was the first time I celebrated a significant event without the participation of my stomach. In my bad old days, I had to stuff my face to have a good time. Unless my belt buckle was digging into my abdomen, I thought I was missing out.

That lifestyle was behind me. One time during the evening, I sat back with a glass of water in one hand and a diet soda in the other. I looked at the wedding party with a fresh perspective. For once, this big fat Greek guy was not pigging out, and that made me feel very thankful.

Monday, May 28
Boston's Fenway Park

Two days after the wedding, I was back on my baseball tour, which, by the way, was going great. In seven weeks I had visited ten ballparks, witnessed thirty-seven games, passed through nineteen states, and driven 6,973 miles.

I took in a classic matchup on Memorial Day—a clash between the Boston Red Sox and their long-standing rival, the New York Yankees. I asked my grandpa John Pfaff to join me at Fenway Park—a ballpark so old that it was cool. Fenway, which opened the same week the *Titanic* sank in 1912, is the oldest major-league ballpark in the country.

It felt good to catch up with Grandpa because my grandmother had died a month before the start of my trip. Grandma's death was a very sad thing. I flew back to Virginia with Mom and carried the casket to her grave. I loved Grandma so much, and she had always been my number one fan, probably because I was her first grandchild. She lovingly teased me. "Nicky, you have to lose weight so you can find a wife," she would say, or "Nicky, you have to lose weight so you can live long and have a relationship with your grandchildren, just like I do with you."

I felt a letdown before the Red Sox game, however. When I performed my weekly weigh-in that morning, the two scales confirmed that my weight loss had gone from a gusher to a steady drip-drip. The weeks of losing seventeen pounds were gone. Now I was shedding a handful of pounds each week. I resigned myself to some tough sledding in the coming months, and I had a feeling that my determination would get called upon in a big way.

Monday, July 2
Seattle

I arrived in Seattle a week before the Major League All-Star game—the Midsummer Classic pitting the best players from the American and National Leagues. I crossed the continental U.S. for the second time in two months, which placed me closer to my goal of visiting all fifty states during my weight-loss trip.

I planned to leave the USS *Spirit of Reduction* in Seattle while I flew to Alaska for a three-day fishing expedition. This side trip would kill two birds with one stone: One, I had never visited the forty-ninth state before, and two, I could go fishing. I love everything about fishing. I love reeling them in, and I love eating them. Fishing was one of the few sports that the morbidly obese could participate in, if you want to call fishing a sport.

When I mapped out my weight-loss trip, I wanted to fish in Alaska during the absolute best, primo time. That would be the month of July, I learned, and when I heard the All-Star game was in Seattle, a plan formed in my mind. Earlier in the year, my brother John and I, along with two of his buddies, booked an Alaskan fishing excursion for July 3–6.

On Monday, July 2, I weighed myself in Seattle, as per my weekly custom. I stepped on both scales, and when I added up the numbers, they came out to 364 pounds. Officially, I had lost 103 pounds since I started my diet on April 1—a ninety-three-day period. That translated into 1.1 pounds of weight lost per day.

While that was a lot of weight, it didn't sound like much to me. When I looked in a mirror, I couldn't even detect a difference in my appearance. I was still wearing the same "Dr. Nick" T-shirts that I wore Opening Day at Dodger Stadium. I had to admit they were a bit looser, but all I saw in the mirror was the same old mound of human flesh. As far as I was concerned, 103 pounds could have been one pound in terms of my visual perception.

I was also bummed because I wasn't losing weight fast enough. Mark Searle, a friend back home, had spent some time programming an Excel spreadsheet for me. All I had to do was enter my weight and the date, and the computer spit out a projection on how much I could expect to lose by a certain date. My goal was to lose 230 pounds, so early on, I harbored expectations that I would reach that lofty ambition by the final out of the 2001 World Series. Now, according to Mark's spreadsheet, I was on track to lose 230 pounds by Thanksgiving—a whole month longer.

On Tuesday, I flew from Seattle to Sitka, Alaska, on a prop plane. Since the Fourth of July was the following day, the Alaskan Airlines flight was full, and I had to endure nearly three hours of in-the-air discomfort.

My miserable mood followed me into Sitka, an otherwise charming seaport village that would be our launching point for three days of fishing. John and his buddies had already arrived, but they were ensconced at the luxurious Kingfisher Lodge overlooking Sitka. They had purchased a package tour that included lodging, meals, drinks— and Happy Hours offering Alaska's freshest and finest seafood!

There was no reason for me to book the same all-inclusive package, so while they were picking at platters of fresh king crab, smoked salmon, and jumbo shrimp before dinner, I quarantined myself at the only budget hostelry in town—the Sitka Super 8 Motel.

Whoopie. I felt like a fat man chained in my own prison while they were partying it up with dozens of fishermen from around the world. My package deal at the Super 8 came with vials of shampoo and conditioner along with directions to the icemaker around the corner. To add to the embarrassment, I had to pack my own blender.

At 7:30 on the first night, John and his friends left their four-star fishing lodge to see how I was doing. I smelled smoked salmon on their breath; they were picking shrimp out of their teeth—and they hadn't been served dinner yet!

"Nick, welcome to Alaska," John said, greeting me with a bear hug.

"Yeah, great," I mumbled.

"Something wrong?" My brother could tell I was in a bad humor.

"Not much is going right. Look at you guys. You're pigging out at the Kingfisher Lodge, and I'm picking my nose in this dump. Even the water tastes disgusting."

"But, dude, we're going fishing tomorrow."

"Like I'll be able to eat any of it. I don't know what I'm doing here. I don't know why I even came to Alaska."

My attitude clearly shocked them.

"No, Nick, you've got it all wrong," one of John's friends insisted. "We're going to have a great time. Just wait and see."

They tried to lift my spirits as we strolled through downtown Sitka, but it wasn't working.

"I'm tired, guys. I'm going to turn in."

I drank a protein shake and retired for the evening long before the sun went down in this land of the midnight sun. Several hours later, around 1 a.m., I was awakened by Sitka's annual Fourth of July fireworks show. Apparently, the local townspeople had a tradition of waiting until it was completely dark to shoot off fireworks. The pounding woke me up, which blackened my mood even more.

I had a wake-up call for 4:30 a.m. As I tossed and turned from the hunger, I wondered how I would handle my first day of fishing. One thing I knew: I was a mess—a tired, dispirited mess.

July 4
Sitka, Alaska

The alarm buzzed at 4:30 on the dot, but I was half awake anyway. It had been a short night, and the lack of sleep bothered me.

While John and his buddies received a ride to the marina, I had to walk fifteen minutes. I felt very sorry for myself—even deprived as I strolled in the early morning mist. I began resenting skinny people. Why were they thin and I fat? What had I done to deserve my fate? During this time of crisis, I even doubted God and His plan for my life.

John and his two friends were waiting at the dock, bubbling with excitement for the first day of Alaskan fishing. My brother said or did nothing insensitive, but I wondered why he was oblivious to what I was going through. *Don't you see my pain? Don't you see the ghetto of emotions I'm in right now?*

The captain boarded the four of us on his boat, a twenty-six-foot Parker fiberglass cruiser with an enclosed cabin and all the latest navigational bells and whistles. The rear of the boat opened up, which gave everyone plenty of room to fish. Kingfisher Charters provided everything: rods, reels, and bait for the fishing and food, snacks, and drinks for the fishermen's stomachs. Just like in Oakland, I was paying for food that I couldn't eat, and that didn't sit well with me again.

It's probably just as well because I got seasick as soon as we pushed off the dock. I didn't have a shake when I awoke at 4:30 a.m., but my landlubber stomach didn't exactly turn me into the captain's pride and joy. I was a maritime wuss, and with each pitch and yaw of the boat, my gills felt as though they were getting greener and greener.

One of the perks of being a physician is that you get to bring along your own stash of meds. I gulped a tablet of Meclizine—an anti-vert that was supposed to take the edge off motion sickness, but that only made me feel drowsy. I was ready to go back to my room and sleep.

As we headed out to sea, the conditions were overcast and breezy. I knew I was in trouble when I saw the wind kicking up frothy white-caps. I glumly looked forward to this day like my male patients looked forward to their annual prostate exams.

Fortunately, we stayed close to shore to fish for king salmon and silver salmon during the morning. Based on my pretrip research, I knew that the king salmon and silver salmon were at their maximum migration patterns. We hadn't set out our lines for more than a few minutes when we got hit after hit after hit. Wow! We kept yanking them in—twenty- and thirty-pounders, right and left, going crazy. The rush of reeling in salmon after salmon put me into pure adrenaline drive, which momentarily caused me to forget my pain and misery. We caught our daily limit of king salmon and silver salmon in less than two hours. (Over three days of fishing, we reeled in twelve hundred pounds of fish. They were cleaned, vacuum-packed, and flash-frozen—four hundred pounds in all. Each of us took one hundred pounds back home, and I ate filets of king salmon, silver salmon, and my prized halibut from December 2001 until July 2002.)

Life was looking up after that rush of excitement. Now it was time to motor into deeper waters to chase the really big fish—Alaskan halibut. The bay had been relatively calm, but once we were out in the ocean, we began bouncing in the chop and whitecaps.

Leaving the safety of the bay was a metaphor for what I was going through with my weight-loss odyssey. My weight had become such a monumental dilemma in my life that I *had* to leave the comfort of the bay and drive toward deep, choppy waters to seek the big catch of a healthy existence.

Fishing for halibut, the captain told us, would be a whole different ball game from trolling for salmon in quiet inlets. He said he would be using his sonar system to find the deepest spots, because the deeper the water, the bigger the fish. "You can catch 'em up to several hundred pounds," he said.

The first few halibut we reeled in were in the twenty- to forty-pound range. They were the biggest fish I had ever caught, but not the Big One. Unfortunately, seasickness grabbed me by the throat again and shook my sensitive stomach. I leaned over the rail, but instead of vomiting, my body shook with the dry heaves. That was a first for me. After ten minutes of the dry heaves, my stomach muscles begged for mercy.

Misery loves company. John became as sick as I was, but he had plenty to throw up—the breakfast buffet and brownbag lunch. Okay, so John and I weren't seafaring Greeks, and perhaps sailing the open seas wasn't in our genes. Then again, the Mediterranean doesn't get too choppy.

There was a mood in the air that said *enough is enough.* It was the captain's call, however, and he had a commitment to keep us out there until two or three in the afternoon. One of John's buddies made a casual suggestion. "Maybe we should head in," he said.

I wasn't ready to give up my fishing pole. Something inside me said, *No, not yet.* "I'm not ready to go," I declared. "I want to keep fishing."

I heard a few groans, but I didn't care. Rain began to fall, so the captain outfitted us with orange plastic canvas parkas, overall bibs, and boots. I was pleased that my rain slicker fit me, although it was a bit snug. I *never* would have fit into that rain gear on April 1. From a distance, though, I probably looked like the world's largest orange M&M.

I looked over and saw John was dying. "Let's get out of here," he moaned.

"No, just a few more minutes," I insisted. I kept working my pole, but I was so weak that I braced myself against the railing. Then, something amazing happened. I had a strike!

My rod bounced off the railing, but I held on tight. "Whoa, I think I've got a big one," I screamed. My rod bent toward the water, and I yanked with all my strength and cranked the reel as fast as I could.

"Steady, steady," the captain advised.

"I'm trying," I said, grimacing. "Whatever's on the end of that line is no normal fish."

I kept dipping the rod and reeling, dipping the rod and reeling. After fifteen minutes of fight, one of John's friends offered to take over.

"Bro, this one's mine," I said, giving the pole another yank, although my arms protested. I was in a dogfight, a war of attrition. The symbolism struck me hard: I was having the fight of my life while I was fighting for my life. This time, I wouldn't give up. The fish would have to pull me into the ocean before I would let go of the pole.

Forty minutes after the initial strike, I reeled the fighting fish to the surface. "It's a halibut!" John yelled out. "A monster."

I knew a fish that big could be dangerous. The way it thrashes around, it could break your leg or damage the boat.

We gaffed the huge halibut and pulled it onto the boat. The monstrosity of the thing! I leaned back against the rail, wowed by the excitement of catching a fish that size.

When the clamor quieted down, I had a question for the captain. "Dave, can you weigh it?"

The captain hesitated. "We don't have a scale that big, Nick."

"So how do you weigh it?"

"You can measure the weight by how long it is."

"Can we do that?"

"Sure," the captain said, who reached for a tape measure. He measured from the halibut's snout to the tail. "It's fifty-nine inches long."

The size of some of the middle-school kids in my practice, I thought.

Dave walked over to the bridge. Next to the steering wheel, he had taped a chart to the wall. He ran one finger down a column, then across . . .

"It's 103 pounds," he announced.

I was stunned. "What did you say?"

"One hundred and three pounds."

The weight of that Alaskan halibut—103 pounds—exactly matched the weight I had lost since April 1. Everything came together for me at that moment because something unspeakable had occurred. It was like I was ushered into the presence of God, who spoke into my heart with an audible whisper, *Nick, look at what you've accomplished to this point. You're going to go all the way.* It was a confirmation of

divine proportions that I never could have expected. Suddenly everything, and I mean everything, made sense. God knew where I was. He
knew everything I was going through. He would be with me the rest
of the way.

A shiver traveled up and down my spine. I had been part of the
most powerful miracle I had ever experienced in my life. Being the
emotional guy that I was, all I could do was cry.

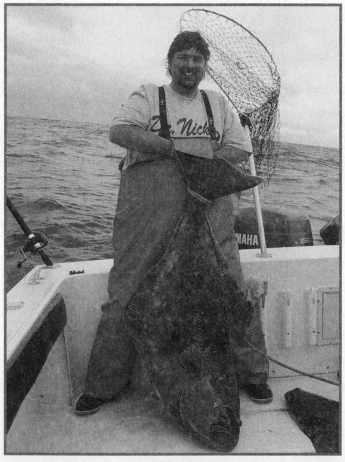

When I learned that my prize catch of halibut weighed 103 pounds—the
exact amount of weight I had lost up to July 4, 2001—I knew I could go all
the way.

John and his buddies slapped me on the back for landing the biggest fish of the day. "Hey, we've got to get some pictures," my brother said, orchestrating a photo op. The fish was so big, though, that I couldn't get a grip on it. Dave suggested tying a rope around its tail so I could lift it off the deck.

As pictures were snapped, I felt the same sense of awe that I felt when I stood in front of Michelangelo's *David* and the Sistine Chapel on a trip to Italy. I couldn't even articulate what was going through my mind, but it was a jumble of bewilderment, love, confirmation, and validation. I knew I had been lifted from the depths of despair. This experience became the deciding moment of my trip, but more than that, the defining moment of my life.

When the New York Yankees bring in closer Mariano Rivera in the ninth inning, hanging on to a one-run lead, Yankee fans know the game's over. When I learned that the halibut weighed 103 pounds, I knew this game was over. I would not be denied after what happened that day.

Even though I had another 127 pounds to lose, that was a formality in my mind. I had tasted victory, and I knew I would be transformed in mind and body into the person I wanted to be.

CHAPTER SIX

FROM THE WINDY CITY TO THE BIG APPLE

Thursday, August 9
Chicago

More Greeks live in the Chicago area than in any other part of the country. Perhaps that explains why I like Chicago so much. I knew the city because I'd spent six weeks in urban Lawndale working at a church-based health center during my medical training days.

With so many old friends to visit, I reserved two weeks in my schedule for the Windy City, which would give me plenty of opportunities to catch a few White Sox and Cubs games. On the diet front, I had passed the halfway point. My latest weigh-in documented a weight loss of 137 pounds, which thrilled me. I was now a one-scale man! I also worked out at several YMCAs in the Chicago area and was actually starting to enjoy exercise. The first time I ever jogged on a treadmill was at the Elmhurst YMCA. I'm sure there's a commemorative plaque marking that achievement.

With less than one hundred pounds to go, I was in the groove.

As for my baseball tour, I attended five games at Wrigley Field, which is what a baseball stadium should be all about. Located in a wealthy neighborhood, the "Friendly Confines" was the last major-league baseball stadium to add lights in 1988, but 90 percent of the games are played when baseball should be played—in daylight. Whenever anyone asks me to name my favorite ballpark out of the thirty I saw, I always reply, "No doubt about it—Wrigley Field."

Wrigley is the only ballpark where your eye is not distracted by a single advertisement or electronic display. Fans are presented a pure, tunnel-vision baseball experience. I soaked it all in—the ivy-covered outfield walls, fans perched in brownstone apartments overlooking Waveland Avenue, and a manual scoreboard updated by attendants swapping cards with each pitch and with each out.

For this afternoon game between the Cubs and the Colorado Rockies, I sat in a great seat right behind home plate, maybe twelve rows up. (Thank you, San Diego Padres.) For a baseball purist like me, a day at the old yard didn't get better than this.

The only bothersome aspect was the oppressive heat. By the time Sammy Sosa hit his first home run of the day in the bottom of the third inning (he would smack *three* round-trippers that day), my sweat-soaked T-shirt stuck to my clammy skin. The Cubs fell way behind the Rockies, and going into the seventh inning, Colorado was up 14–4. I didn't care. The traditional seventh-inning stretch in the bottom of the inning was coming up, and I loved singing "Take Me Out to the Ballgame" at Wrigley.

I was sucking on my third or fourth diet cola when—out of nowhere—I heard a woman's high-pitched scream. I turned around and witnessed a middle-aged woman, three rows behind me, shriek a second time.

My medical instincts, which had been dormant for nearly five months, immediately kicked in. The fastest route between two points is a straight line, so I jumped over three rows of seats to discover an older woman slumped in her seat. "I'm a doctor," I said, taking control of the situation. "What's wrong?"

"It's my—my mother," the woman blurted.

I pressed my right index finger to the woman's carotid artery in her neck, searching for a pulse. Then I leaned my face closer to hers, looking for evidence of respiration. There was neither. This woman, who looked to be in her seventies, was dead.

Instinctively, I sprang into action. "Move! I'm a doctor," I shouted to the stunned fans seated in her row. "Get out of the way!" I lifted the dead woman into my arms and gently laid her on the concrete.

I was about to start CPR when an usher came running up. "We need to get her out of here," he said. "There's a game going on."

I didn't even look up. "Get lost. This woman is dead. She's not going anywhere."

I initiated CPR with a cardiac thump, which is a brisk pounding against her chest. It's a technique that works only when the cardiac arrest is attended to within seconds. When there was no response, I initiated the pumping action of CPR, which came back to me as naturally as tying my shoelaces.

After two cycles of CPR, as is the custom, I paused and put my cheek against her face and my fingers against her carotid artery. With astonishment, I heard gentle respiration and detected a faint pulse. Her eyes popped open and met my gaze. "I'm thirsty," she said.

This woman would live! I had witnessed another miracle. I firmly believe that God allowed me to be at the right place at the right time to help this woman start breathing again.

Several minutes later, paramedics arrived. I barked out a summary of what had transpired as they inserted an IV into her arm, attached a monitor to her chest, and efficiently put her on a backboard and carried her out of the ballpark.

As I got up from my swollen knees, something very strange happened. I received an ovation from the Cubbie faithful seated in the home plate area. I sheepishly raised my hand in acknowledgment while I returned to my seat, trembling with incredulousness at the divine moment that had just occurred. My excitement was tempered by the sobering thought that I had been used as the hands of God.

I hadn't been settled long in my seat when some guy four rows back bellowed, "Doctor, that was amazing." I swiveled my head to thank him. Then in true baseball hospitality fashion, he yelled out, "Yo, Doc, can I get you a beer?"

How touching. "Thank you, but I don't drink," I said, almost laughing.

The man was persistent. "Doc, well, then let me buy you a hot dog."

At which point in time, I didn't know what to say, so I told him the truth.

"I don't eat either," I said with a shrug of the shoulders.

He looked at me as if I were from another planet. Within earshot of dozens of Wrigley fans, I had no choice but to explain who I was and what I was doing.

I did not even get a chance to watch the last two innings of that game. For the next half hour, I told my story—the one you've been reading about in this book—to a group of mesmerized, disbelieving Wrigley Field fans. *Going around the country watching baseball games while drinking protein shakes?* It couldn't be true. I could tell by their expressions that they were having great difficulty believing me.

Some of the Cubs fans suggested that I talk to someone from WGN, the Chicago superstation found on many cable TV systems around the country. I demurred. I wanted my story told in the right way at the right time.

One thing I knew: It would be hard to top what happened at Wrigley Field.

September 10
Cooperstown, New York

The National Baseball Hall of Fame is the shrine to baseball's greatest players, a repository of artifacts that include everything from Babe Ruth's locker to Sammy Sosa's bat when he hit his five-hundredth home run. I visited the Hall of Fame with my grandfather on September 10, and all I can say is that it was an absolute assault on my baseball fan's senses.

I lived in Greece between the ages of four and nine, and when we returned to the United States, I was so happy to be back in America. I love this country. When we arrived on U.S. soil during the midseventies and resettled in New Jersey, the Yankees were back on top. I got swept up in the excitement of a pennant chase and World Series; these were the "Bronx Zoo" days with Reggie Jackson and Billy Martin. Ever since then, I've made a connection between America and baseball, and perhaps that's why I love this country and adore this game.

I certainly felt the connection in Cooperstown, a precious, tender, quaint town in upstate New York. I told Grandpa that I could spend another day at the Hall of Fame, but I had tickets for the baseball game the following night, September 11, at Yankee Stadium.

Grandpa and I hopped into the USS *Spirit of Reduction* and drove Route 17 to Mahwah, New Jersey, located on the north end of Bergen County. Mahwah is a bedroom community for New York City.

As we pulled into the driveway at the house of my cousin Terry Mostyn that evening, I was bummed that I couldn't see Manhattan's distinctive skyline—the World Trade Center, the Empire State Building, and the Chrysler Building—that I was so familiar with as a child. *No big deal,* I told myself. I would see the skyscrapers on my way to the Yankee game the following afternoon.

September 11, 2001
Mahwah, New Jersey

"Nicky, Nicky! Something's wrong! A plane just crashed into the World Trade Center!"

Whoa. Where was I? That sure sounded like my grandfather talking to me. What was he so agitated about? I had never heard him that way. It had to be another one of those weird dreams.

Then I felt my body being shaken. "Wake up, Nicky. You have to see this on the TV!"

I cracked open my eyes. "What did you say, Grandpa?"

"It's on the TV! Look!"

My grandfather turned on the small TV in my guest room, and from the first image, it looked bad. The north tower of the World Trade Center was billowing in smoke. The CNN news team was saying that a passenger jet had mysteriously struck one of the Twin Towers.

It didn't seem possible. No passenger planes flew that close to the city on their way to JFK or LaGuardia.

Grandpa and I couldn't believe our eyes. A few minutes later, we gasped when we witnessed a second plane ram the South Tower—live on TV! I had never been stunned like that in my entire life. I was convinced that the world was coming to an end. I sat transfixed as I watched flames and smoke envelope the Twin Towers, and I felt sickened that hundreds, probably thousands, of innocent people were trapped in the upper floors.

Desperate souls were jumping left and right out of the towers when suddenly the South Tower collapsed! The sight of a 110-story building imploding on the Manhattan landscape tripped the same altruistic feelings I felt at Wrigley Field. I had to get involved.

Oh, my gosh . . . oh, my gosh . . . With trembling hands, I picked up my cell phone and called the Escondido Community Health Center. It was a little after 7 a.m. on the West Coast, and I knew that Carol, one of the administrative assistants, always came in early.

"Carol? Dr. Nick here," I said. "You've seen the horrible news?"

She had. "Listen, I need you to fax my credentials right away. I want to go into New York. Perhaps I can be of some help." I assumed that Lower Manhattan resembled a war zone, and able-bodied physicians would be needed. "Let me give you the number of my cousin's fax machine. It's . . ."

My grandpa and I threw some of my belongings into the van and sped toward the George Washington Bridge. We listened to the radio as the North Tower collapsed. A few minutes later, we turned a corner, and I could see the swelling pillars of smoke emanating from Manhattan.

While I feverishly drove, I also worked my cell phone. I called and offered my medical assistance to the Red Cross, the New York Medical Society, and every trauma center in the area, including the hospital where I was born in Englewood, New Jersey. I desperately wanted to help out. Because this is where I grew up, I identified with everyone I saw that fateful day.

We drove to Hoboken, located directly across the Hudson River from Manhattan. I witnessed ferry boats discharging hundreds of numbed people covered with ash and soot. Nearby, refugees by the thousands were streaming on foot across the George Washington Bridge. I parked close to the bridge and showed a cop my medical credentials and asked if I could walk into New York City, but he prevented me from doing so.

I had an excellent contact—a good friend named Dr. Willy Foster, who was an emergency room doc in the Bronx. I called his home, expecting to talk to his wife, but Willy answered the phone.

"What are you doing home?" I asked.

"I'm on call, Nick, but there's no one coming in. I don't think there are many injuries."

A sickening sense of doom fell over me. I realized there would be many deaths but few injuries that day. I was deeply disappointed because part of me felt that I was born for that day. I had anticipated jumping into the front lines, saving lives and aiding the injured. I felt like I was wired to respond to catastrophic situations like this, but that would not be the case on September 11. My medical skills were not needed.

I had to do *something*, though, and my chance came three days

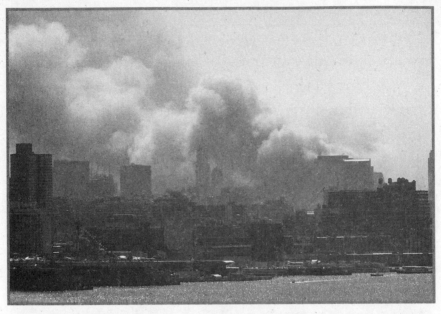

I took this photo on September 11, 2001, and I was an eyewitness to a world changing before my very eyes.

later on Friday, September 14. My cousin and I drove to Manhattan, and while we understandably couldn't get within blocks of Ground Zero, I volunteered to counsel at the armory near Gramercy Park, which had been converted into a center for grieving family members. The sight of hundreds standing outside the armory, holding pictures and hoping for word of their relatives or friends was one of the most gut-wrenching experiences of my life. I patiently listened to many of them, bleary-eyed from grief and worry, tell their stories of the last time they had heard from their loved ones, or the last-minute phone calls they received from those trapped in the upper floors of the burning Twin Towers. Some clung to the hope that their loved one lay in a burn unit, alive but unidentified.

For all too many, it was hope against hope. For me, September 11 was a grim reminder that each day is precious—and a gift from God. This event renewed my determination that once I reached my weight-loss goal, I would do whatever it took to stay there.

It's sad how it took a tragedy of this magnitude to shock many in our country back to the realization of what life is all about. Life is a gift, a gift we cannot take for granted, and certainly a gift to which we should provide nothing but the greatest of care. As a result of this experience, I had a renewed sense of appreciation for my personal health and the commitment I now had to be a good caretaker of it.

CHAPTER SEVEN
MAKEOVER DAY

November 9
Bedford, Virginia

My grandfather John Pfaff lived in Bedford, a Civil War town with nineteenth-century storefronts and gracious manor homes dating back to the 1830s. When I arrived to see him for a few days, he informed me that his friends in the local senior citizens group wanted to hear about my weight-loss odyssey at their next weekly meeting. Oh, and a newspaper reporter from the *Bedford Bulletin* would be there, too.

When I stood up in front of three dozen senior citizens, let me tell you, I was shagging some hair. My brown curly locks spilled past my shoulders, and I must have looked like a WWF wrestler to them; all that

85

was missing was a black Speedo. I could tell these oldsters were think-ing: *Yeah, right, he's a doctor.*

You may have already thumbed through the pictures of me in this book and wondered what the deal was regarding my long hair. Well, I've always loved how symbolism can apply to the truth of our daily existence, and for me, my hair took on symbolic significance. When I was a child, I was enthralled by the story of mighty Samson, a man of superhuman strength. I had cartoon books of Samson that I read and reread before I turned off the lights at night.

Samson was set apart by God for a special purpose—to rescue Israel from the Philistines. His mother was instructed to never cut his hair, and he grew up known for feats of strength: He ripped a roaring lion in half, single-handedly killed a thousand men, and broke ropes as if they were spiderwebs. What Samson accomplished was because of God, and his long hair publicly symbolized that God-given strength.

Way before I started my weight-loss trip, a thought came to me: *To accomplish my rather audacious weight-loss goal, I would have to be dependent on God's strength working through me.* I already knew what I was capable of accomplishing on my own—ballooning up to 467 pounds with a sixty-inch waist was evidence of that. When I decided to turn my life around, I knew I would have to be utterly dependent on God's strength, so I symbolically made a public pledge to my family and friends that I would not cut my hair until I accomplished my goal.

When I arrived in Bedford, I had lost 204 pounds, and now my weight was 263 pounds. I only had twenty-six pounds to go. As far as I was concerned, the end was in sight. I made the decision to go home with a triumphant splash, but I had no idea that lopping off my locks would empty the pool.

Now, there's something you should know, especially if you are not obese. For most of my adult life, I attempted to hide my weight and who I really was. For instance, I would often put on an extra layer of clothing, as if that would be effective in hiding my double-wide trunk. I sported a goatee or beard, as if facial hair could disguise my face's bloated features. My days of hiding behind a mask were over.

On November 9, I visited the Bedford Science and Technology Center, which included a cosmetology institute, which is a fancy name for "haircutting school." The woman in charge raised her eyebrows when I asked for one of the students to go to town on me.

I was escorted to a gum-smacking young woman I'll call Jenny, who looked to be around eighteen years old. She motioned me to her styling chair.

"What's your pleasure?" she asked.

"I want to go from looking like an unemployed, homeless NFL lineman to a member of a boy band."

To her credit, she was game. "NSYNC or Backstreet Boys?"

"Just do me, girl."

She needed specifics, so I listed them:

- Snip off my long hair.
- Leave me with a spiked cut, real tight.
- Make me a blond.
- Shave off my goatee and mustache.

The novice hairstylist was blown away. "No way. You're like serious, right?" Jenny asked.

"*Beaucoup* serious," I replied. "Jenny, there's one other thing. I want to donate my hair to a child with leukemia, so if you could cut off the maximum amount, that would be great."

"Cool," she said.

Several strategic snips produced a sixteen-inch lock of hair that was lovingly bundled at both ends with rubber bands and placed in a storage bag that I would later send to a charitable group called Locks of Love. That symbolism of strength would be woven into a wig that would be given to a child with leukemia who had become bald from chemotherapy treatments.

For the next three hours, I became the focal point of a roomful of teeny-bopping, chitter-chattering eighteen-year-old girls. I sat in my chair thinking, *Hmm. It feels good to get a little physical attention for something besides my skin folds and waistline.*

Jenny, to her credit, mustered all her budding cosmetic skills on my makeover. The hair left on my dome was spiked and bleached with hair color, turning my dark brown hair to a harvest-yellow thatch. Then she foamed up my face and took a straightedge razor to my goatee. When she was done, I saw raw skin on my chin for the first time in a decade.

When Jenny spun the chair around for my first good look in a mirror, I barely recognized myself. I'm sure you harbored the same thought after seeing my before-and-after pictures.

For fun, I added a magnetic stud earring to my left earlobe, and *voilà,* my physical metamorphosis was complete. I knew I would freak out a lot of folks when I returned to my grandfather's house that afternoon. I was right. My relatives' children, who had waved good-bye to me that morning, didn't recognize me!

The following week, I departed the East Coast for my sixth continental crossing. My "Take a Swing at Weight Loss" tour was winding down. I had taken in 109 baseball games, attended the last four World Series games between the New York Yankees and Arizona Diamondbacks, hopscotched my way through forty-nine states, and added more than thirty-seven thousand miles to the odometer of the USS *Spirit of Reduction*. Now I was going home again, and it sure felt good.

Thanksgiving 2001
Escondido

They say the biggest travel day of the year is the Wednesday before Thanksgiving. I was on the road, too, urging the USS *Spirit of Reduction* to find its way back to home sweet home. The traffic headed south Wednesday afternoon on Interstate 15 was heavy, but more people seemed to be *leaving* San Diego than going into America's Finest City.

Throughout my eight-month weight-loss odyssey, three San Diego media outlets had been tracking my progress—the *San Diego Union-Tribune*, the *North County Times*, and KUSI Channel 9. Reporters stayed in touch via e-mail or called my cell phone. I had never sought media attention or hired a publicist, but when they heard I was coming home for the Thanksgiving holiday, they all wanted to be in on the story.

Ed Lenderman, a KUSI news reporter, had aired several stories on me during the year. When I told him about my homecoming plans, he asked if he could meet me a couple of exits before my freeway off-ramp and follow me to my house. I said no problem.

With a KUSI news truck in my rearview mirror and a cameraman in my van, I pulled onto our street only to see a gaggle of reporters, photographers, and other media types milling about my family's front yard. I had warned Mom that there could be a few photographers when I arrived, but I wasn't prepared for anything like this. I also asked Mom and the extended family to wait in the house until I knocked on the door. I love good surprises, and I wanted to *really* surprise Mom and Dad, my siblings, my in-laws, and assorted nephews and nieces when I stepped through the front door.

What happened next was like a Publisher's Clearinghouse moment. A group of reporters, cameramen, and grips formed a tight circle as they followed me to the front door. I knocked, and when Mom opened the door, she cupped her face in utter surprise. What transpired in the next sixty seconds was a mixture of confusion, bewilderment, and excitement as evidenced by the shrieks of Mom and the other family members who rushed to the door. They were shocked by my appearance, and for good reason. I had brought home only 249 pounds and undergone a dramatic makeover that changed my appearance in a huge way.

My nephews and nieces—all preschool age or younger—ran crying into their mothers' arms when I tried to pick them up. They didn't recognize who this "Uncle Nick" character was! The only little members of the family who recognized me were my pet Chihuahuas. They licked my face and greeted me like a long-lost friend.

I like to tell people that what happened that afternoon was a Visa moment:

Tickets to 109 major-league baseball games: $7,243
2,800 gallons of gas to drive all over America: $4,290

Purchasing the USS *Spirit of Reduction* and all other travel expenses: $17,734

The look on Mom's face when she opened the door and first saw me: PRICELESS!

Thanksgiving Day

KUSI Channel 9, a UPN affiliate, reaired the three-minute piece of my homecoming four or five times that day. My homecoming story also landed on page one of the *North County Times* and page one of the *Union-Tribune's* local section.

Not everyone reads the papers, of course. That morning, I ran into several neighbors, and they regarded me with confused looks. "Do I know you?" several asked. Others commented, "You sure look familiar." I could have been part of a federal witness protection program.

"It's me—Nick, Dr. Nick," I would say, and their look of confusion quickly gave way to one of wonderment and surprise. I could feel their joy and their enthusiastic response to my transformation. Doris Warren, one of my longtime elderly patients, had to be propped up after she got a good look at me. The poor thing nearly fainted.

KUSI and several other media outlets, including the region's two largest newspapers, asked if they could hang around the Yphantides Thanksgiving dinner and capture the moment—the big moment— when I would eat my first bite of solid food since the Last Supper back on March 31.

Don't get the wrong idea. I wasn't falling off the wagon. Although I was just twelve pounds from my weight-loss goal, I knew that sooner or later I would reintroduce real food into my diet. The idea of eating with my extended family on Thanksgiving Day—remember, I'm a guy who loves symbolism—sounded great to me. Thanksgiving is my favorite day of the year because it's the only American holiday not caught up in the hype and commercialism that surrounds Halloween, Christmas, and Easter. Thanksgiving is a time of fellowship with those you love and an opportunity to thank God for the tremendous blessings He's bestowed on you in the past year. That's why home and hearth were calling me for the Thanksgiving holidays.

Thanksgiving dinner was held in the early afternoon at my brother Phil's house. We gave camera crews and photographers permission to film the clan—numbering two dozen—preparing the turkeys (one was dipped into a deep-fat fryer!) and grilling the portobello mushrooms and zucchini on Phil's back patio.

Our family had no intention of altering our Thanksgiving routine of giving thanks to God just because of the presence of TV cameras. We carried on the family tradition of standing around the main table holding hands, united in heart and spirit as we sang the Doxology— *Praise God from whom all blessings flow . . . Praise Him, all creatures here below . . .*

Dad then offered a heartfelt prayer, thanking God for the tremendous way He had protected us and provided for us in the past year, including my safe arrival home. As I listened to Dad's voice crack with emotion, I felt deeply humbled at the miracle God had wrought within me.

We sat down, and all eyes—plus TV cameras—immediately pointed in my direction. In a few moments, I would eat real food—not food I would have to drink—but food that required a knife and a fork to bring it to my mouth. As mundane as this habit is for billions of people around the world, I had been deprived of this routine for nearly eight months. My teeth, missing in action for eight months, had been called up for active duty.

I had carefully chosen—after some medical consultation—what I would eat on Thanksgiving Day. My digestive system could tolerate only soft, mushy vegetables after such a long sabbatical. Had I eaten a slice of turkey breast and stuffing—animal protein and fats—right off the bat, I would have faced the risk of nausea, abdominal cramps, and a gallbladder attack. Solid food had to be introduced in a very gentle manner. Like a prisoner locked for months in a pitch-dark dungeon, I needed to be gradually reintroduced to the sunlight of solid food.

With a flourish that would make a maître d' blush, my sister-in-law Betsy set before me a plate of her finest china decorated with a splendid display of mouthwatering food. In the center of the plate sat the main entrée—a small baked potato stuffed with eggplant purée surrounded by a grilled portobello mushroom, a dab of spinach, a pair of sliced tomatoes decorated with rosemary leaves, and two orange wedges. Talk about presentation!

I have to tell you, though, I had a mixed reaction to seeing a plate of food set before me. My mind was so dialed in to *not* eating that I was reluctant to reach for my fork and knife. Another thought was that the last time I ate, mushrooms, spinach, sliced tomatoes, and potatoes were mere accoutrements to the *really* good-tasting food found in meats, cream, and cheese.

Although I would be eating a vegetarian meal, there was a little ham in me once the cameras began rolling. I took my fork and knife—I hadn't held those utensils in a long time—and cut a piece of portobello mushroom, piping hot from Phil's barbecue. I set that small slice of mushroom into my mouth, and suddenly my gastric juices sprung to life like the Old Faithful geyser. Wow, that tasted good! It was a truly culinary orgasmic moment, one that I hadn't experienced since I let the last bite of banana cream pie melt in my mouth.

I arched my back as an ecstatic energy burst through my body, and I kept going with it: I fell backward to the floor and landed in a heap, only to quickly pop up with a football-wide grin on my face.

For the next four weeks, I slowly reintroduced food groups into my diet while I continued to drink one or two protein shakes a day. Culminating with more symbolism, I enjoyed my first bite of meat on Christmas Day—a slice of succulent turkey breast. Those bites of turkey tasted so good that I felt I had been born again on the day our family celebrated Christ's birth.

Early 2002

After arriving home, I sold the USS *Spirit of Reduction*, dealt with the mountain of mail, started working twenty to twenty-five hours a week at the medical clinic that I used to direct, and devoted two to three hours a day at the YMCA to keep that weight off.

When the Yphantides family rang in the New Year, I was within a few pounds of reaching my weight-loss goal of 230 pounds. It looked like I would weigh 237 pounds sometime during the first week of January. That's when I decided to shoot for a new weight: 210 pounds. This would mean losing twenty-seven more pounds.

You know me: I love a challenge, and I gave myself a goal of reaching 210 pounds by April 1, the one-year anniversary of my weight-loss odyssey. Before April Fools' Day rolled around, though, I also had some unfinished business. I had one more state to visit—Hawaii!

A buddy, Jon Petersen, and I rectified that oversight by flying to Honolulu during the last week of March. Something interesting happened before the long flight over the Pacific Ocean. Upon boarding, I found my seat in economy class, settled in for a moment, and then I pushed the call button for the flight attendant. I did that without thinking because when I had flown before, I needed the flight attendant to bring me a seat-belt extension.

Then I remembered: I no longer weighed 467 pounds. I tried to buckle up without the seat-belt extension, and lo and behold, my lap belt not only fit, but I had three or four inches to spare.

"Can I help you, sir?" the flight attendant inquired.

"Ah, no, ma'am. Sorry about that."

I had never been to Hawaii before. I mean, why would a walrus lie on the beach? But Jon and I had quite a time hanging out at Waikiki Beach, snorkeling at Hunama Bay, and eating roast pig at an authentic Hawaiian luau.

I didn't eat a huge quantity of roast pig, but for the first time in the last year, I enjoyed more than the sights when I was on the road: I also got to sample the *tastes* of the local culture. Think about it: When I visited New Orleans and the French Quarter during my weight-loss odyssey, I couldn't dine on Creole gumbo. When I passed through Kansas City, I couldn't eat barbecue. When I breezed into Chicago, I couldn't eat a slice of their famous deep-dish pizza. When I stopped in Bridgeport, Maine, I had to shake my head no to all that crab and lobster.

For all the deprivation I had experienced, Hawaii rekindled an appreciation for the importance of food as a pleasant way to enjoy the culture. Another highlight was the simple joy of going to the beach without covering up from head to toe.

Jon and I returned home a couple of days before April 1, and you know by now that April Fools' Day is a significant date for me. On April 1, 2000, I set my weight-loss journey in motion when I formally notified the Escondido Community Health Clinic that I would be leaving April 1, 2001, to embark on my weight-loss journey. I've detailed what happened that day when I stepped on two scales and learned—to my horror—that I weighed 467 pounds, one hundred pounds more than expected.

When I stepped on the scales April 1, 2002, I had reached my second weight goal: 210 pounds. I had officially lost 257 pounds. I took a nostalgic look at the photo taken one year earlier of my naked, plump, oversized body. In 365 days, I had become less than half the man I used to be.

September 2002
Mount Whitney, California

I continued to lose weight during the summer of 2002, and the day after I climbed 14,495-foot Mount Whitney—the tallest peak in the contiguous United States—I reached my official weight-loss nadir: 197 pounds.

When I began my incredible journey, I couldn't have followed a climbing team up a flight of stairs without begging for mercy. For Mount Whitney, I completed a five-day, fifty-mile hike like it was a walk through the park.

I've since gained fifteen pounds, but that's from working with weights that added muscle mass to my body. Now I'm just trimming the sails and trying to maintain a steady course. One thing I know: I'm never going back to 467 pounds.

Perhaps you're morbidly obese like I was. Maybe you're packing a good-sized tire around your midsection. Maybe you could stand to lose twenty pounds.

I don't care where you are or what you weigh. You can do it. For the rest of this book, I'm going to show you how you can change your life so that you can change your weight. In addition, I'll present "Dr. Nick's Seven Pillars," which will enable you to make major changes in your life.

This is not the end.

This is only the beginning.

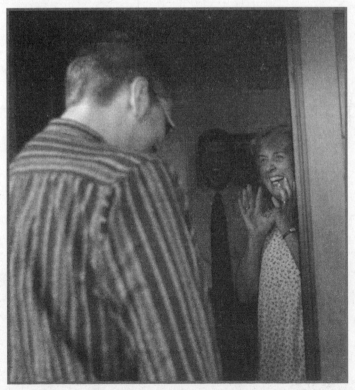

The local news media was there when my mom opened the front door and saw me for the first time in nearly eight months—more than 230 pounds lighter.

PART II

MY BIG FAT GREEK DIET

DR. NICK'S SEVEN PILLARS

CHAPTER EIGHT
THE SEVEN PILLARS OF WEIGHT LOSS AND MAINTENANCE

I know what you're thinking: *That's an entertaining story, Nick, but what about me? I've been overweight for a long time. I need some hope here—and a lot of help.*

If that's the way you feel, stick with me because in the rest of the book, I plan to gush forth a veritable fountain of advice and encouragement. My weight-loss principles, which I call "Dr. Nick's Seven Pillars," will give you a framework within which to change your life so that you can change your weight.

I know what you're thinking again: *C'mon, Nick. You're not turning this into another one of those boring diet books, are you?*

Ever since my weight-loss story captivated the San Diego media during 2001, the publicity has churned up dozens of invitations to speak throughout California. For several years running, I've regaled audiences large and small with a PowerPoint presentation hitting the high points of the story you just read. But I've quickly learned that overweight people are hungry for something more than just my feel-good story. They are eager to devour information that will start them down the right road. "What can I do to lose weight, Dr. Nick?" they ask. "I'm desperate. I've tried everything. Please help me!"

I'm wired to help people become healthy—I took the Hippocratic oath, remember. I developed the Seven Pillars because I've always been captivated by the number seven. In the Greek culture, the notion of the Seven Wonders of the Ancient World can be traced back to the Greek author Antipater of Sidon, who lived in the second century BC. He settled on seven because the Greeks considered that a symbolic number. (I chose the word *pillars* because it conjures up memories of the powerful stone columns I saw when I visited the Parthenon in Athens, where I spent my early childhood.)

Seven is also said to be God's number for perfection. From the seven days of creation to the seven seals of Revelation, the Bible is saturated with the number seven or multiples of it. Jesus said we are not to forgive others seven times but "seventy times seven."

For some of you, this may be the 490th book you've read on losing weight, but I hope it's your last. *My Big Fat Greek Diet* can be, if you'll adopt the principles behind my Seven Pillars. I'm confident you'll be receptive because I'm writing from the perspective of a medical physician who's personally lost hundreds of pounds. That's an unusual combination in the saturated world of diet books. The famous doctors who've authored diet books—such as Dr. Robert Atkins (*Dr. Atkins'*

Diet Revolution), Dr. Arthur Agatston (*The South Beach Diet*) and Dr. Phil McGraw (*The Ultimate Weight Solution*)—never had to step on two scales to determine how much they weighed. They never heard the schoolyard taunts of "Bacon Boy" or "Lard Butt." They never walked a day in size EE shoes.

I lived with obesity for twenty years, and the feelings of emotional pain and humiliation are as fresh today as they were leading up to the Last Supper. I'll never forget the cruel comments from kids and the looks of disgust from adults. One time I walked into an examination room to see a three-and-a-half-year-old girl who had a fever. Before I could even open my mouth, Amy proclaimed, "My doctor so fat, Mommy! Why so fat, Mommy?"

"You shush, Amy," the mother said, as embarrassed as I was. "That's not nice to say to our doctor."

I smiled weakly, but inside I was dying. For the entire visit, I remember being distracted and devastated. I kept saying to myself, *From the mouths of babes.* But the mouths of adults—even relatives—could be just as hurtful and ruthless in their criticism of me. I can recall a holiday occasion when a well-meaning but blunt-talking Greek aunt cornered me and poked a finger into my chest. "You should be ashamed of yourself," she spat. "It's disgusting for a doctor to be so fat!"

That's why I can feel your pain. You've been the target of similar barbs, and there's been nothing you could say in your defense. You've told me so. I've hugged folks just like you after I've spoken before audiences and community groups. I've cried with obese patients who felt life wasn't worth living. I've comforted grieving family members after they suddenly lost an obese father or heavyset mother prematurely to a heart attack.

Those who aren't fat have no idea what it's like to live in a culture where thin people are celebrated by the media, given starring roles in films and TV series, and—dare I say it?—get the promotions at work. Seventy percent of television characters are thin, according to one survey, while just 5 percent are overweight. Our culture holds up supermodels as ideals of fashion and glamour, but their weight and measurements are light-years away from the build of the average American woman.

What a mixed-up society we live in. On one side, we have an epidemic of young women so obsessed with their weight that they develop eating disorders such as anorexia nervosa and bulimia. On the other hand, we have a growing population of overweight and obese individuals unprecedented in human history. "Americans are the fattest people on Earth and getting fatter every year," a Harris interactive poll announced. Harris, which has been researching the numbers of overweight Americans for more than twenty years, says that 58 percent of Americans were overweight in 1983, 64 percent in the early 1990s, 71 percent in 1995, and 80 percent today. This upward trend mirrors what I see in the trenches of my medical practice every day.

Why are we getting fatter? Because we're eating more and exercising less. I mean, *Duh.* I believe Americans are consuming more food and more calories because we're eating more meals away from home—in restaurants where food is fried, breaded, buttered, and drenched in artery-clogging sauces. In 1955, the average American family spent 25 cents of their food dollar in restaurants. Today, 46 cents of every food dollar goes straight into the cash registers of McDonald's, Taco Bell, Chili's, and Cracker Barrel. Time, pressure, convenience, marketing campaigns, and the widespread availability of fast food all make this understandable. Because competition for the American food dollar is so intense, restaurants serve heaping portions so the American public thinks it's getting a good deal.

Sit-down restaurants aren't taking the "burger wars" lying down. Their toque-hatted cooks stack mashed potatoes into a mountain resembling the Matterhorn and cut slabs of prime rib into sixteen-ounce hunks that a caveman would have appreciated. Even the salads are humongous; a single serving could feed a high-school football team. The typical bowl of lettuce and greens comes loaded with meat, cheese, croutons, and fat-heavy dressings, which defeats the purpose of eating a "healthy" salad.

Between meals, we're tempted in food courts, airport terminals, and stadiums to indulge our sweet tooth. High-fat, high-sugar treats like Cinnabons, Dairy Queen Blizzards, and the mega-popular Starbucks Frappuccinos (the chocolate brownie version has 510 calories and 22 fat grams) are available on every corner of the country.

VAST IMPLICATIONS

The fact that our government classifies two-thirds of American adults as overweight carries all sorts of health-care implications. Overweight people see the doctor more often and are hospitalized in greater numbers due to higher rates of life-threatening conditions such as diabetes, coronary heart disease, and other serious chronic ailments. Almost 80 percent of obese adults have at least one serious complication. A study by RTI International and the Centers for Disease Control and Prevention, published in the *Journal of Obesity Research*, shows that the nation is spending about $75 billion a year on weight-related diseases. Health-care costs for illnesses resulting from obesity now exceed those related to both smoking and alcohol abuse. About 325,000 deaths a year are attributed to obesity.

Health-care insurers are raising premiums to cover their increased costs, which are then passed on from employer to employee. This will only get worse and indirectly contributes to the growing number of people in our country left without private health insurance. About half of the $75 billion yearly price tag for obesity is covered by tax-payers in Medicare and Medicaid programs.

These days, newspapers and newsmagazines are peppered with stories or feature articles presenting a fresh angle or the latest research regarding our growing "obesity problem." I'm glad that obesity is on front pages and magazine covers because the alarm bell should be sounded. The number of extremely obese American adults—those at least one hundred pounds overweight—has *quadrupled* to four million since the 1980s. In the past, one out of every two hundred adult Americans was morbidly obese; now it's one out of every fifty.

What *really* shocks me is the rapid growth of severely obese people—the fattest of the fat . . . folks who would have been my twin when I started my weight-loss trip. According to a study performed by *The Archives of Internal Medicine*, people with a BMI (body mass index, which I'll explain soon) of fifty or more grew from one in two thousand in 1986 to one in four hundred in 2000. A typical man in that group stands five feet ten inches tall and weighs 373 pounds. Get that man another scale!

And get that man some help. That's why I've devoted a great deal of thought to developing my Seven Pillars. I'm confident that you'll find them practical, realistic, and applicable. My bedrock principles can be summed up this way:

DR. NICK'S SEVEN PILLARS
OF WEIGHT LOSS

I. Change the way you see before you change the way you look. Fundamental to addressing one's health issues is addressing the cause. Permanent weight loss is impossible without a permanent lifestyle change.

II. Slash your calories by eating for the right reasons. Why we eat and how we eat are more important than what we eat. Learning why and when to eat and how to stop eating at the right time is key.

III. Fill your tank with the right amount of the right foods. Diets do not work. Eating the right foods the right way does.

IV. Burn calories like never before. Weight reduction and maintenance are impossible without sustained and vigorous physical exertion. The muscles of your body are designed to be used.

V. Plan a radical sabbatical. There is magic in combining doing something you love with something that is great for your health. I call it the "distraction from deprivation."

VI. Don't travel alone. The path to a healthy life cannot be accomplished solo. Being accountable to others and putting it on the line with others are essential.

VII. Realize that your weight-loss journey is for a lifetime. Losing the weight is not the real issue. Keeping it off and never finding it again is.

In the next seven chapters, I'll expand on each concept and show you how to apply the Seven Pillars to your life. Following that are chapters that discuss:

- Fast food and our meals-on-the-go culture
- What parents can do to help their obese children lose weight
- The hot new trend of gastric bypass surgery

Now that I've given you the road map of where we're going, we need to do an attitude check.

FOLLY AND WISDOM

When I weighed 467 pounds, I was a young man who overate, underexercised, and expected to enjoy a normal life expectancy. That's how foolish I was. Yes, I said *foolish,* and that's why I started my weight-loss odyssey on April 1. April Fools' Day will always carry enormous significance for me, and it is now my personal holiday—the Fool's Thanksgiving.

Looking back, I wonder what took me so long to make this major lifestyle change. I was a medical doctor, for goodness' sake, a family physician in his early thirties who cared for hundreds of overweight and obese patients each month. Few were in the pink of health. In fact, I could predict what ailed them from the moment I stepped inside the examination room:

- Diabetes
- Hypertension
- Heart disease
- Degenerative arthritis

I knew the root cause of their illnesses—they weighed too much. But did I ever connect the dots and say to myself, *Nick, if you don't make a change, this is your destiny, buddy?*

I may have, but if I did, I didn't let my mind go *there*. That's because I was a fool. Then the light flipped on when someone shared the following advice:

Fools do not learn from their mistakes and experiences.
Smart people learn from their mistakes and experiences.
Wise people learn from the mistakes and experiences of *others*.

Are you going to learn from my mistakes and experiences? I hope so, because I was traveling through life as foolishly as my overweight patients were, maybe even more so because I advised them about what diet they should go on! I know that the mental image of a 467-pound doctor patiently explaining the pros and cons of the Atkins' diet, *Mastering the Zone,* or the grapefruit diet doesn't compute in your consciousness, but that's what I did every day at the Escondido Community Health Center. At the end of every consultation, though, I cleared my throat and smiled. "Don't forget: Do as I say, not as I do," I said.

"Sure, Dr. Nick. Whatever you say."

My patients were receptive because I projected this Jolly St. Nick image of a larger-than-life physician who cared for their well-being and their future health in a big way. When I ran for public office in 1996 for a position on the Palomar Pomerado Health Board, my campaign slogan was "Big Problems Need Big Solutions. Vote for the Big Man, Dr. Nick." You probably knew that I would say this, but I won by a landslide.

I snowballed the competition because my patients and my community knew I cared about them and sought to give them the best health care. Whenever overweight people came to see me, they quickly learned that I was well read on the popular diets and could address their upsides and downsides with authority. I could even speak from personal experience because I had tried many myself. Whether it was the cabbage soup diet, fasting, or the Atkins' diet, however, I failed miserably every time. I often found myself losing a few pounds (this was back in the days when I weighed less than 350 pounds) before growing discouraged and chucking another diet into the dustbin. Then I quickly returned to my bad old ways and regained those pounds, plus some more.

Nobody has dieted the first eight or nine hours of the day more often than I have. No matter how good or how strong my intentions were, however, by mid-afternoon my stomach was growling like a demented wolf pack. To satisfy the munchies, I binged on a package of DoubleStuf Oreo cookies (a package of twenty-eight cookies had 1,960 calories), or I asked an office assistant to pick me up a carne asada burrito—make that two burritos with extra cheese and sour cream—at a nearby taco shop. I might have satisfied the hole in my stomach, but I didn't satisfy the hole in my heart.

The weight-loss industry was built on the backs of people like me. It's universally agreed that 95 percent of all diets fail, which only keeps overweight people coming back to the Diet and Health section at

Barnes & Noble or ordering some new gadget or "bun-cruncher" via an 800 number. The amount of money shelled out on weight-loss products, weight-loss programs, and medical intervention tops $40 billion annually, according to Marketdata Enterprises. That's $109 million per *day*. Much of this money is spent on programs and gimmicks that don't get to the heart of the issue. Weight-loss companies are telling people what they want to hear, not what they *need* to hear.

The reason overweight people throw so much money at the weight-loss industry is that we want to lose weight *today*. Yesterday would be even better. This explains why we reach for our wallets when viewing infomercials touting "eight-minute abs" or George Foreman grills that "knock out" the fat. Here are some of the outrageous claims you'll hear:

- **"Lose weight while you sleep."** Anyone can lose weight while he or she is sleeping. That's because they're not eating! Unfortunately, it's what you eat while you're *awake* that determines what you weigh. That doesn't stop charlatans from peddling pills that "cause your body to burn fat while you sleep."
- **"Lose all the weight you can for just $99."** I've seen flyers posted on telephone poles in my neighborhood, and they are come-ons to buy prepackaged meals, sort of like Jenny Craig. I have nothing against heating up a Weight Watchers or Jenny Craig frozen meal, but it's going to cost a lot more than $99 to follow those programs.
- **"Eat as much as you want, exercise as little as you want, and lose five to ten pounds a week—guaranteed!"** You usually see bold claims like this in tiny ads in magazines that breathlessly

proclaim a "scientific breakthrough" and a "medical miracle" that could "save your life!"

- **"This miracle pill is all you need!"** I remember the time— before I lost all my weight—when an obese woman asked me whether there was *something* I could prescribe for her. "Don't you have anything that could help me lose weight, Dr. Nick?"

Remember, I was way over four hundred pounds in those days. "Let me ask you something," I said in my best Jolly St. Nick persona. "Let's say there was a medication that was safe and effective to lose weight. You get only one guess. Who would be the first person taking that medication?"

"Ah . . . that would be you," she said.

"And there's your answer."

I had this conversation a thousand times if I had it once. Hey, I would have *loved* to prescribe myself a "fat pill" and wake up thin the next day or thirty days later or six months later. But as I've learned over the years, you can't take pills to lose weight, just as school kids can't swallow a "smart pill" so they don't have to study in school.

You would be foolish to believe any of these claims. If it sounds too good to be true, it definitely is, as Mom always told me. That hasn't stopped the pharmaceutical industry from trying to develop legitimate drugs that treat obesity. They are doing tons of research in an earnest attempt to discover new prescription options.

Currently, physicians can prescribe only two drugs for long-term therapy: Xenical, which reduces dietary fat absorption; and Meridia, an appetite suppressant. In clinical trials, both drugs produced only a 5 percent to 10 percent loss of initial body weight. Like many medications, Xenical and Meridia have potentially serious side effects such as increased heart rate and diarrhea. These drugs have proved to be effective only when taken in combination with a comprehensive weight-maintenance program. I have never prescribed these drugs for two reasons: Many of my uninsured patients cannot afford them, and I'm not convinced of their safety and efficacy. Let's put it this way: I wouldn't have taken them myself when I weighed 467 pounds, which means I could never prescribe them to one of my patients.

Let me end this chapter with this thought: Don't be foolish like I was. King Solomon, the wisest man who ever lived, once wrote, "Wisdom has built her spacious house with seven pillars" (Prov. 9:1 NLT).

Seven pillars.

I can relate to that, so keep reading and become wise by learning something from this formerly fat fool.

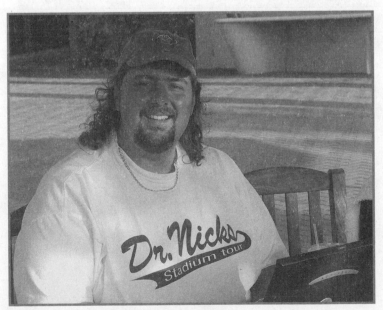

I would have been a big fat fool if I hadn't taken a swing at weight loss.

CHAPTER NINE

PILLAR I:
CHANGE THE WAY YOU SEE BEFORE YOU CHANGE THE WAY YOU LOOK

Remember *Kojak*, the cop show from the 1970s? Telly Savalas—my favorite Greek actor of all time—sucked on a lollypop and said, "Who loves ya, baby?" Well, who loves you? I'm sure your family does. Your friends, too. Even some of the people you work with. They love you. They want to see you change your life.

I was reminded of who loved me—and whom I loved—when I was stricken with testicular cancer. I fought for my life because I didn't want to leave my family and close friends behind. But if that life-threatening event had never happened, I'd possibly weigh more than five hundred pounds today. Sure, I would have been bummed that I weighed so much, but I would have felt stuck and figured nothing could have been done about it. When I was confronted with my mortality, I came to the stark realization that my physical life was precious. I had to change the way I saw my life so that I could change the way I look.

My hope is that it will not take cancer or something that drastic to spark a similar epiphany in your life. Don't wait until you have a heart attack. Don't wait for the doctor to announce that you have diabetes. Don't wait until your gait slows to a shuffle and you're addicted to pain medication for deteriorating joints.

I'm sure you're not in a hurry to die. So what more do you need to be convinced that being healthy is the essence of living? Don't you have enough to look forward to—taking trips with friends, watching your children grow up, living to a ripe old age? I want children and big fat Greek weddings for my sons and daughters. I guess I'm so Greek that I'm already thinking about grandkids.

The incentive to change must come from deep within. My appreciation for life deepened after having cancer and facing my mortality. I rediscovered the valuable gift that life really is; for me, it is a personal gift from a loving God who cares deeply about every aspect of my existence. It has become my life's desire to love God in return by caring for the gift of health that He has given me. Without some level of appreciation for this truth, losing weight and becoming healthy would, for me, become a futile exercise. It is the very core of my motivation.

The vulnerability that allows people to fall prey to ridiculous infomercials, bogus magazine advertisements, and overhyped programs is a result of desperate people trying to lose weight for the wrong reason. I'm talking about something different. It's like you've been given just one car to drive for your entire life. How are you taking care of that car? Running it into the ground by eating midnight snacks? Pumping the wrong fuel into the tank? Failing to maintain the U-joints and other moving parts?

The motivation to lose weight should be to live a better life, not to look better. Remember, people, this is not just about losing weight. This is about losing weight and keeping it off. This is about losing it and never again finding it. This is about losing weight and having no idea where you put it.

Rick Warren, in his best-selling book *The Purpose-Driven Life*, expressed thoughts similar to mine. He also said that to change your life, you must change the way you think. He used this word picture to explain himself:

> Imagine riding in a speedboat on a lake with an automatic pilot set to go east. If you decide to reverse and head west, you have two possible ways to change the boat's direction. One way is to grab the steering wheel and physically *force it* to head in the opposite direction where the autopilot is programmed to go. By sheer willpower you could overcome the autopilot, but you would feel constant resistance. Your arms would eventually tire of the stress, you'd let go of the steering wheel, and the boat would instantly head back east, the way it was internally programmed.
>
> This is what happens when you try to change your life with willpower. You say, "I'll *force* myself to eat less . . . exercise more . . ." Yes, willpower *can* produce short-term

change, but it creates constant internal stress because you haven't dealt with the root cause. The change doesn't feel natural, so eventually you give up, go off your diet, and quit exercising. You quickly revert to your old patterns.

There is a better and easier way: Change your autopilot—the way you think . . . Change always starts first in your mind. The way you *think* determines the way you *feel,* and the way you feel influences the way you *act.* ([Grand Rapids: Zondervan, 2002], 181–82)

Changing the way you see is like changing your autopilot. Rick is 100 percent right: You can't force yourself to become slim by saying, "I think I can, I think I can," like the Little Engine That Could. Instead, you must change the way you see yourself and your excess weight before you can change the way you look.

TWO FUNDAMENTAL TRUTHS OF WEIGHT LOSS

Just as you didn't become overweight overnight, you won't necessarily shed weight very quickly. I lost an incredible average of 1.1 pounds per day by utilizing an aggressive protein shake diet. Unless you do something drastic like forsaking solid food for a while (and that's okay for some), you shouldn't expect to lose more than one to three pounds per week. This will vary widely, depending on multiple factors, including one's age and sex. Keep in mind that many diets promise—and induce—large amounts of weight loss the first week or two by flushing the body of valuable water, but merely losing "water weight" means that the pounds will quickly come back once you resume eating your usual foods. You're not accomplishing much by doing intermittent short-term diets, no matter how aggressive they are.

The excess weight hanging on your frame is a symptom that something is fundamentally wrong with your life. Whether you have a spare tire weighing twenty or thirty extra pounds or you're dragging the equivalent of two American women with every step as I was, you need to be aware of two fundamental truths:

1. You are putting more energy into your body's engine than it needs.
2. You are burning less fuel than your body is designed for and capable of burning.

When you're overweight or obese, you're overflowing your tanks at every pit stop and not driving very far between fill-ups. Your body is not designed to be "topped off" with extra fuel when it doesn't need any. Your body is designed to run efficiently with just enough of the right fuel in the tank.

Storing extra fat is like putting extra storage tanks in the back of your pickup. You're lugging more weight, which prompts you to eat more to keep those tanks filled. You're slowly killing yourself in the process. Your biological vehicle is bound to break down and need a medical mechanic like me to get you back on the road again. Here are the common diseases and medical health issues you can expect to deal with as you lug around your excess weight:

- **High blood pressure/hypertension.** Bodies with extra weight put an extra burden on the heart to generate more pressure to keep the tissues nourished. High blood pressure catches up with you, and in the long term, weakens the heart by forcing it to work harder than it should.

- **High cholesterol and fat.** Overweight people are more likely to have elevated levels of bad cholesterol and fat circulating in their blood vessels. Our cholesterol level is an important internal indicator of our nutritional health. There is a "good" kind of cholesterol called HDL, which carries circulating fat away from the tissues. We want that number to be as high as possible. "Bad" cholesterol, called LDL, carries and deposits fat in the body's tissues, and we want that number to be as low as possible. Your doctor can easily check your cholesterol levels and interpret what your numbers mean.

  Elevated levels of bad cholesterol increase the likelihood of blockage forming in arteries, thereby limiting blood flow to vital organs. When a blockage prevents blood from reaching the heart muscle and causes muscle death, we call it a heart attack. When the blockage prevents blood from feeding a part of the brain and causes partial brain-tissue death, we call it a stroke. When the blockage prevents blood flow to the tip of a limb, leading to the death of skin and soft tissues, we call it gangrene.

- **Diabetes.** Excess fat tissue can limit the body's ability to respond to its own chemicals. Excess fat decreases the body's sensitivity to its own insulin. Insulin is a vital hormone that regulates and maintains circulating sugar levels. The decreased sensitivity increases the insulin and sugar levels in the body, leading to the syndrome of diabetes with its host of medical complications.

- **Gallbladder disease.** It is a well-known fact that patients who are obese have a much higher risk of developing gall-stones, gallbladder attacks, and the digestive complications associated with them.

- **Arthritis.** Our joints are not designed to survive the additional pounding that comes with carrying around so much excess weight. Degenerative arthritis of the knees, hips, and ankles is an inevitable consequence for the obese. It becomes a vicious circle: Debilitating pain limits activity, which increases weight, which increases pain, which limits activity even more, which adds even more weight.

  When I began my weight-loss odyssey, my knees were shot. I already have radiologically documented degenerative arthritis. For the three years leading up to the Last Supper, I was dependent on non-narcotic anti-inflammatory medication to make it through each day. After losing weight and taking hundreds of pounds off my knees, I still hear crunch and crackle sounds whenever I sit down. The damage has been done. One day, I will be required to have surgical replacement of both knee joints. Being fit will help postpone my destiny with the surgeon's scalpel as long as possible.

- **Sleep apnea.** For some of you, snoring may be pathological enough to be labeled an illness. Sleep apnea is a serious, potentially life-threatening condition that is characterized by brief interruptions in breathing during sleep. The risk of sleep apnea increases when weight gain, especially in the throat and neck area, causes the excess tissues around the breathing passages to compromise respiratory function. The condition owes its name to a Greek word, *apnea*, which means "want of breath."

As a fat man, there was nothing I enjoyed more than lying down in bed and escaping the realities of my existence with a good night of sleep. Other than stuffing my face, sleep was my number two recreation. The problem was that you didn't want to sleep in the same room with me when my eyelids shut for the night. People who lived to tell about the experience said I sounded like a lumber mill. I dreaded church retreats or occasions when I shared a hotel room with someone. I always packed a set of earplugs in my shaving kit, but they weren't for me. I usually offered them to the luckless person who drew the shortest straw and had to sleep in the room with me.

I will never forget the men's retreat where I was assigned to the bottom bunk in a cabin with twenty-four beds. (Can you imagine a 467-pound man climbing up to the top bunk? I could have killed someone if that upper bunk splintered under the force of my weight.) I must have snored like Chris Farley on the first night because I remember how one of the guys sheepishly approached me the following morning.

"Listen, Nick, after last night, I was wondering . . . wondering if you would be willing to sleep in the lobby."

"Lobby?"

"Yeah, the lobby. They have a couch in there."

Ouch.

I couldn't blame the fellow. My snoring emitted a loud, vibrating, groaning reverberation of sound. So many people complained that I knew I had a serious problem. One night, I taped myself with a recorder to self-diagnose my snoring patterns—something I asked my patients to do when I suspected sleep apnea. What I heard the following morning shocked me. My snoring intervals got faster and faster, but then my breathing suddenly stopped for a while. That was classic sleep apnea, which scared me. What if after one of those long pauses, I didn't resume breathing? I knew as a medical doctor that breathing patterns and the low oxygen levels were wrecking havoc on my heart and lungs. If your snoring knocks photos off the night-stand, or your spouse comments about momentary pauses in your breathing cycle while you're asleep, you'll definitely want to discuss this with your doctor.

Sleep apnea, which afflicts eighteen million overweight Americans, is serious stuff. It wasn't that long ago that people died in their sleep. Today, many obese patients require special pressure-generating breathing machines just to survive through the night.

- **Asthma and chronic bronchitis.** The inflammatory process that occurs in the lungs is made worse by excess tissue around the lungs pressing on the chest wall cavity. Overweight people are more likely to wheeze and struggle to breathe, which limits their exertional capacity.
- **Cancers.** Conclusive evidence suggests that obesity increases the risk of certain types of cancer, including breast, prostate, colon, and endometrial, among others. The cause and effect of why cancer strikes some individuals are complex and not completely understood. Some blame cancer on the obesity

itself, while others believe lifestyle choices put one at higher risk for these cancers.

- **Emotional pain.** I don't need to remind you about the anguish that your excess weight causes to your psyche. Obese children are so down in the dumps that they rate their quality of life on par with children being treated for cancer with chemotherapy. University of California researchers compared quality-of-life scores of obese children with those of normal-weight children and determined that the obese children were nearly six times more likely to report an impaired quality of life.

I can speak from personal experience. For as low as I felt when I submitted to cancer radiation therapy in my early thirties, it did not compare to the deep emotional anguish I experienced as an obese person. The pain in my heart is gone now, but I can still vividly recall it. With regard to the other harmful effects of obesity, thankfully I have been blessed with good genetic wiring. While my blood pressure and sugar and cholesterol levels were on the edge, I never reached a point where I required medical treatment. Other than my crunchy knees, I made the drastic changes early enough in life to avoid suffering other irreversible consequences.

REALITY THERAPY

Have you been spending years looking for the Fountain of Skinny? I'm talking about a figurative river of magic with such miraculous curative powers that if you bathed in its waters, you'd instantly turn into a *Baywatch* babe or a studmuffin with rock-hard abs.

The Fountain of Skinny doesn't exist, but that hasn't stopped millions of overweight folks from chasing after a certain pill, the right diet, or the newest tummy flattener for what ails them—excess weight. Weight loss doesn't happen that way. I realized that there was no way I could drastically change my weight without totally changing my life. Change had to begin internally. Like Dorothy's desire to return to Kansas in *The Wizard of Oz*, the power to change the way I looked had been within me my entire life.

You can click the red ruby slippers as well. My suggestion is that you find a quiet place soon—today, if possible—where you can't hear the TV, can't see a computer screen, and won't be interrupted by loved ones or work colleagues. You need to clear your head and think about what you want to do with the rest of your life. How long are you going to remain overweight or obese? Ten years? Why can't it be five years then? If five years, what's stopping you from making a one-year commitment as I did? Have you had it? Are you at the end of your rope?

At the end of the day—or your life—you and only you can answer the following fundamental question:

What do you have to do to change the way you see before you can change the way you look?

Once you've made up your mind to change the way you see things, then you can start thinking about a plan to change the way you look. I plan to talk about the pros and cons of various diets later, but let me state that you will have to change your eating habits. (Sorry, no getting around that.) You will have to exercise. You will have to learn to eat for the right reasons. You will have to plan on committing six to eighteen months to reach your weight goals. You will have to devote a lifetime to maintaining them.

To start, you need to know from where you'll begin your journey. Do you have a few pounds to lose, which means only minor adjustments need to be made? Or do you have more than one hundred pounds to lose, and major changes in your life must occur? If I were seeing you in my examination room, I would start off with some assessment tools to determine your starting point.

For most doctors, the standard gauge of one's size is the body mass index, or the BMI. The BMI uses a mathematical formula that takes into account a person's height and weight. As a strict formula, the body mass index equals a person's weight in kilograms divided in height in meters-squared. I grew up with meters and kilograms in Greece, so the metric system works for me, but I understand we talk in feet and inches and pounds here in the U.S.

To the right, I've provided a converted body mass index table using inches and pounds. Just find your height in the left-hand column and run your finger across the columns over to your height. The row above your weight (a number between 19 and 54) is your BMI. (You can also go to healthsteward.com and calculate your BMI there.)

Here's a breakdown of what the BMI numbers mean:

- 18 or lower: underweight
- 19 to 24: normal
- 25 to 29: overweight
- 30 to 39: obese
- 40 to 54: extremely obese

BODY MASS INDEX TABLE

Body Weight (pounds)

Height (inches)	Normal						Overweight					Obese										Extreme Obesity														
BMI	19	20	21	22	23	24	25	26	27	28	29	30	31	32	33	34	35	36	37	38	39	40	41	42	43	44	45	46	47	48	49	50	51	52	53	54
58	91	96	100	105	110	115	119	124	129	134	138	143	148	153	158	162	167	172	177	181	186	191	196	201	205	210	215	220	224	229	234	239	244	248	253	258
59	94	99	104	109	114	119	124	128	133	138	143	148	153	158	163	168	173	178	183	188	193	198	203	208	212	217	222	227	232	237	242	247	252	257	262	267
60	97	102	107	112	118	123	128	133	138	143	148	153	158	163	168	174	179	184	189	194	199	204	209	215	220	225	230	235	240	245	250	255	261	266	271	276
61	100	106	111	116	122	127	132	137	143	148	153	158	164	169	174	180	185	190	195	201	206	211	217	222	227	232	238	243	248	254	259	264	269	275	280	285
62	104	109	115	120	126	131	136	142	147	153	158	164	169	175	180	186	191	196	202	207	213	218	224	229	235	240	246	251	256	262	267	273	278	284	289	295
63	107	113	118	124	130	135	141	146	152	157	163	169	175	180	186	191	197	203	208	214	220	225	231	237	242	248	254	259	265	270	278	282	287	293	299	304
64	110	116	122	128	134	140	145	151	157	163	169	174	180	186	192	197	204	209	215	221	227	232	238	244	250	256	262	267	273	279	285	291	296	302	308	314
65	114	120	126	132	138	144	150	156	162	168	174	180	186	192	198	204	210	216	222	228	234	240	246	252	258	264	270	276	282	288	294	300	306	312	318	324
66	118	124	130	136	142	148	155	161	167	173	179	186	192	198	204	210	216	223	229	235	241	247	253	260	266	272	278	284	291	297	303	309	315	322	328	334
67	121	127	134	140	146	153	159	166	172	178	185	191	198	204	211	217	223	230	236	242	249	255	261	268	274	280	287	293	299	306	312	319	325	331	338	344
68	125	131	138	144	151	158	164	171	177	184	190	197	203	210	216	223	230	236	243	249	256	262	269	276	282	289	295	302	308	315	322	328	335	341	348	354
69	128	135	142	149	155	162	169	176	182	189	196	203	209	216	223	230	236	243	250	257	263	270	277	284	291	297	304	311	318	324	331	338	345	351	358	365
70	132	139	146	153	160	167	174	181	188	195	202	209	216	222	229	236	243	250	257	264	271	278	285	292	299	306	313	320	327	334	341	348	355	362	369	376
71	136	143	150	157	165	172	179	186	193	200	208	215	222	229	236	243	250	257	265	272	279	286	293	301	308	315	322	329	338	343	351	358	365	372	379	386
72	140	147	154	162	169	177	184	191	199	206	213	221	228	235	242	250	258	265	272	279	287	294	302	309	316	324	331	338	346	353	361	368	375	383	390	397
73	144	151	159	166	174	182	189	197	204	212	219	227	235	242	250	257	265	272	280	288	295	302	310	318	325	333	340	348	355	363	371	378	386	393	401	408
74	148	155	163	171	179	186	194	202	210	218	225	233	241	249	256	264	272	280	287	295	303	311	319	326	334	342	350	358	365	373	381	389	396	404	412	420
75	152	160	168	176	184	192	200	208	216	224	232	240	248	256	264	272	279	287	295	303	311	319	327	335	343	351	359	367	375	383	391	399	407	415	423	431
76	156	164	172	180	189	197	205	213	221	230	238	246	254	263	271	279	287	295	304	312	320	328	336	344	353	361	369	377	385	394	402	410	418	426	435	443

Source: Adapted from Clinical Guidelines on the Identification, Evaluation, and Treatment of Overweight and Obesity in Adults: The Evidence Report.

I guess I would have been off the chart because the standard BMI Index table doesn't even have my old weight of 467 pounds. Leave it to Nick to set a dubious record.

Things are looking a lot better today. I stand 74 inches tall (that's six feet two inches), and my current weight is 210 pounds. To find my BMI, my finger searches for number 74 in the left-hand column and slides over to the 210 box, which tells me that I have a BMI of 27. That makes me overweight according to the BMI, but I have more muscle mass these days since I hit the weight room several times a week. Remember, the BMI tool is an estimation, not an exact science. In some quarters, the BMI has been criticized for misclassifying people because of their muscle mass.

Other assessment tools can supplement the BMI in determining personal body weight goals. I like the simple formula in which you count one hundred pounds for the first five feet of height of a woman, then add an additional five pounds per inch for every inch over five feet. That gives you a ballpark estimate for her ideal body weight.

For example, the ideal weight for a five-foot five-inch woman would be 125 pounds using this formula, although I must point out that this tool does not take into account skeletal frame size, muscle mass variations, and even unique curveballs such as the weight of her breast implants. (I see a lot of those in San Diego, which has to be the cosmetic surgery capital of the world.)

For men, the equivalent equation is 110 pounds for the first five feet of height, and an additional six pounds for every inch above five feet. Using this formula, a six-foot man's ideal body weight would be 182 pounds. For someone my height, 194 pounds would be my "ideal" weight.

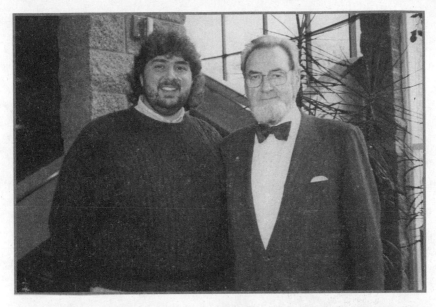

As a physician involved in public health care in San Diego, I've been fortunate to rub elbows with former Surgeon General Dr. C. Everett Koop and (bottom picture, from the left) Elias A. Zerhouni, M.D., director of the National Institutes of Health, Julie Gerberding, M.D., director of the Centers for Disease Control, Mark McClellan, M.D., former Food and Drug Administration commissioner, and Richard Carmona, M.D., U.S. Surgeon General.

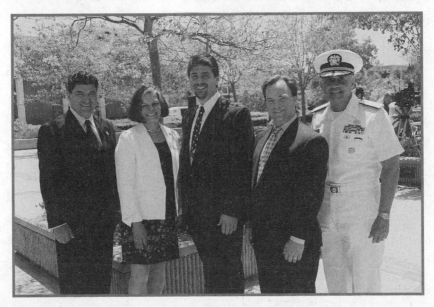

As I mentioned, these calculations do not take into account the important body frame variations—specifically the size and width of your bones. A basic but not entirely accurate way of determining your skeletal size is to grasp one of your wrists with the thumb and index finger of the opposite hand. If your fingers do not touch, you're a big-boned person with a large frame. If your thumb and index finger just meet, you have a medium frame. If they overlap, you have a small frame. My thumb and index finger don't come close to meeting, so I have a large body frame, which partly accounts for the extra sixteen pounds I carry.

In the long run, these assessments are merely a snapshot of where you are right now. I think it's important to document where you are *before* you start changing your weight so that you can be encouraged to press on during the ups and down of changing the way you see yourself. That's why I did my weigh-in with my brother Phil. We needed a baseline so I could measure whether I was going in the right direction.

You have to be honest with yourself. Don't be like a compulsive gambler—lying to yourself and others while underestimating your weight. To become healthy, lose weight, and keep it off, there has to be a change—a change of lifestyle, a change of behavior, a change of thinking, and a change of perspective.

We are all unique individuals created by God, which confirms what I saw in my practice: There cannot be a one-size-fits-all mentality regarding weight loss and personal fitness. The changes necessary for one to lose weight and achieve optimal health must be customized. For those of you who have less weight to lose, the degree of change may not be that complicated. You may need to create more time to be physically active. Maybe you need to go to a soup-and-salad restaurant instead of a taco shop for lunch.

I don't think successful weight loss and maintenance are possible without at least some degree of change. How deliberately you are willing to do this is something only you can know. For me, the way my perspective has changed since 2001 has rocked the core of my existence. I've gone from being a workaholic to a lifeaholic who works just enough to put salad on the table. I've gone from taking my health for granted to understanding that waking up each morning is a gift from God. I've gone from someone who was in denial regarding the consequences of my weight to someone enthusiastically eager to make the most out of every waking moment. Losing weight is not about a temporary fix; it's about having a new perspective and a new motivation. It's about a new approach to life in the way we think, the way we eat, and in the way we use our bodies. I had to change the way I saw things before I could ever change my weight.

I've gone from eating various forms of processed and preserved food and plastic-wrapped junk to enjoying the taste of food in its natural and original form. I've gone from being a couch-dwelling creature to someone who's an active and enthusiastic exercise machine. I've gone from eating to deal with my pain and loneliness to eating to satisfy my physiological hunger. I've gone from packing my stomach to the point of discomfort to learning that it's good to leave the table feeling appropriately satisfied. Food has gone from being a centerpiece of my existence to being one of the many things I love and enjoy about life. I used to live to eat, but I now eat to live, as you'll see in my next pillar.

CHAPTER TEN

PILLAR II: SLASH YOUR CALORIES BY EATING FOR THE RIGHT REASONS

September 29, 1997, is a date that will live in infamy for me. That afternoon, I received confirmation that I had testicular cancer. Although the prognosis was good—"Nick, I think we caught it in time," my urologist said—I suddenly realized that perhaps saving for retirement was something I could scratch off my to-do list. The idea that I could actually die took on the force of brute reality, which shook me to the core. What lay ahead was the surgical removal of my right testicle, followed by nearly three months of intensive radiation. After that? My doctor didn't give me any ironclad guarantees. My life was in the hands of God.

I managed to maintain my composure in the doctor's office, but once I got behind the wheel of my vehicle, I sobbed like a child who had lost his mother. I wiped away salty tears so I could read the stoplights and make out stop signs. I groaned in pain and cried out to God to save my life. I couldn't pull myself together even as I pulled into my parents' driveway. When I stepped inside the front door, family members greeted me with a look of fear, seeing my devastation as their own tears began to flow. Others spoke in hushed tones. Some guarded their comments, but few looked me in the eye. It was like attending your own funeral.

The extended family had quickly assembled inside my parents' living room, including my mother, my three brothers, and my sister, Pauline, along with assorted in-laws. My father was in New Jersey at the time, visiting his siblings and extended family. After the initial awkwardness, word spread, and within minutes we were receiving emotional calls of concern from all over California, the East Coast, and even Greece.

The focused attention was getting to me. "I'm going out for a ride," I mumbled to Mom. "I need some fresh air." I slipped out the front door and wedged myself behind the steering column of my Expedition. I didn't need fresh air, however; what I needed was something to eat. Whenever the chips were down, food lifted my sagging spirits. Whenever I had scored poorly on an important medical school test, was turned down for a date, or ridiculed for my size, I always found solace with my very best friend—a plate of warm food.

Food loved me unconditionally, and that love had gotten me through many dark times. This time, the storm clouds gathering around my life had never been blacker. On this gloomy afternoon, I knew just the place to go—the KFC restaurant on Broadway Avenue, where Colonel Sanders's bearded visage would be waiting to greet me like a long-lost friend. KFC had been the delicacy of choice for my family growing up. I can still remember singing the KFC jingle in the car with my brothers while we were on our way to share a bucket of the Colonel's best.

I walked up to the counter and ordered a five-piece extra-crispy dinner, which came with mashed potatoes, gravy, corn on the cob, and two biscuits. I carried my plastic tray filled with the KFC value meal to an empty table. I took my time setting out my box of chicken and various side dishes in preparation for this holy sacrament of eating. I bowed my head and returned thanks to the Lord, and then I picked up one of the Colonel's chicken breasts, personally cooked by him. Taking a long look at the double-breaded skin coated in eleven secret herbs and spices, my mouth watered in anticipation. Then I took my first bite, slow and easy, since I didn't want to rush this culinary experience. My food returned love when I needed it most. With each chew of fried chicken and each forkful of mashed potatoes, I received another helping of emotional comfort.

It almost makes me physically ill to recount this story because in my most vulnerable moment of my life, I had left the people who loved me more than anyone in this entire world for a box of fried chicken and several side dishes. That's how strong a hold eating had over me. It wasn't until I had forsaken solid food for eight months that I learned how wrong it was for me to believe that only food could soothe the anguish and pain in my heart. I was no better than Esau, the Old Testament character who sold his inheritance to his brother Jacob for a single meal of bread, peas, and stew.

I know that I didn't eat at KFC that day because I was hungry. I ate to satisfy a hole in my heart, not to satisfy a hunger in my stomach. Quite simply, I ate for the wrong reasons, which all overweight and obese people do to varying degrees. To lose weight effectively, you will have to learn how to eat at the right time for the right reasons, which is the foundation point of Pillar II.

I ate at KFC because I was emotionally distraught, and emotional eating is one of the Seven Traps of Eating. (I know, the number seven again.) Let's take a closer look at some of the inappropriate reasons people overeat:

TRAP #1: EMOTIONAL EATING

Do you eat when you're depressed? Do you eat when you're lonely? Anxious? Stressed? Preoccupied? Angry?

I ate for all the above reasons. I've known men and women who, after having been romantically rejected, masked their emotional pain by turning to food. Some smother painful early life experiences—verbally abusive parents, emotionally negligent abuse, or even sexual abuse—by ordering a large stuffed-crust pizza to be delivered to their front door. Maybe your emotional pain started when you were an adolescent and classmates mocked you at school. After you carried that burden home with you, Mom soothed you with cookies and milk.

Roadside diners pride themselves on serving "comfort food"— meatloaf, country-fried steak, macaroni and cheese, and chicken potpie. They know their market—lonely truckers far from home, single-parent moms struggling to get by, and down-and-outers look-ing to pass the time. Their motives for eating can be linked to emotional reasons. We've all been there at one time or another. Any trauma or reality that causes unpleasant feelings can prompt us to inappropriately deal with it by eating our way out of the blues.

TRAP #2: MINDLESS EATING

Prior to losing my weight, I hosted a Super Bowl party every year for my family and friends. Around twenty-five to thirty people usually showed up, but I always had enough food on hand to feed one hundred football fans. Every Super Sunday, my mother said, "You're putting out enough food to feed a Greek army. The teams aren't coming this afternoon—your friends are."

The reason I prepared so much food was to show my friends how much I loved them. Out here on the West Coast, the pregame shows start at noon, which is a long time before the 3:18 kickoff. This gave us plenty of time to graze the finger foods and fill a plate or three with slices of turkey breast, piles of cheese, and chips and dips. We kept eating from the opening kickoff to the spectacular halftime extravaganza, throughout the thrilling second half, and into the champagne-soaked postgame show. That adds up to seven hours of mindless munching.

Have you ever engaged in this form of reflex eating? Sure, we've all nibbled on snacks and goodies because "they're there." This form of eating is not in response to hunger. We absentmindedly reach for the bowl of chips, the wedge of jalapeño cheese, or the green beans wrapped in bacon with nary a thought as to *why* we're eating.

I never thought about why I ate when I was growing up. Whenever somebody came over to visit, the food had to come out. You couldn't come to our house and not have something to eat— that's not how *koinonia* works. It was like when my dad and I visited those Greek friends near Pebble Beach during the first week of our trip. Our families barely knew each other, but when we stepped inside their house, it was like a conveyor belt was positioned between the kitchen and the dining room table. "I just made some fresh *tiropita!* You must try a piece," the matriarch said. In my bad old days, I would have tried the fresh cheese pie even if Dad and I came straight from a restaurant. Why? Because it was being offered to me.

We're such gullible people. Have you watched couples at the movies? They buy a tub of greasy popcorn, a box of Milk Duds, and a liter of Coke. This happens twenty minutes after they finished eating dinner in a restaurant!

Mindless eating happens every day in the workplace. You pass the break room, where someone has left something to snack on, so you instinctively grab a handful of nuts, chomp a few crackers, tear off a piece of bagel, or crack a doughnut in half. You're not hungry, and the food may not taste particularly fresh or even good, but it's there for the taking (and it's free!), so you graze.

TRAP #3: RECREATIONAL EATING

Out here on the Left Coast, we have "foodies." They dine in the finest restaurants and think nothing of spending $100 or more on an evening of sybaritic self-indulgence. They rhapsodize over the filet of red mullet covered in a sauce made with aged scamorza, debate the merits of cauliflower served in a cream of chestnuts and topped with white truffles, and reach the heights of culinary decadence with a *filet de boeuf* topped with quail egg, a timbale of cardoons, and a tortellone of fonduta.

Foodies are always flocking to the hot restaurant, watching Emeril on the Food Network, and occasionally cooking up a storm in their

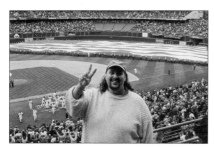

2001 Major League Baseball Opening Day

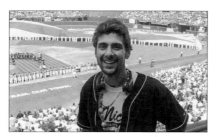

2002 Major League Baseball Opening Day

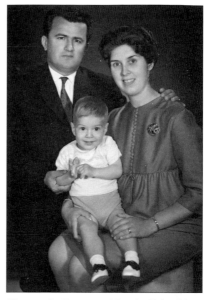

My parents, George and Bernice Yphantides, didn't overfeed me, although I would be later told to clean my plate "because your father worked hard for this food."

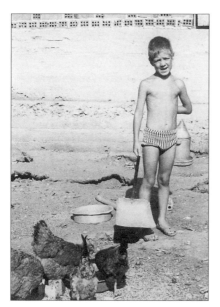

I wasn't an obese kid growing up because I was constantly outside playing. Here, I investigated chickens as a young boy growing up in Greece.

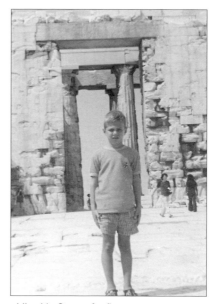

I lived in Greece for five years as a young child, where our family went on outings to the Parthenon in Athens.

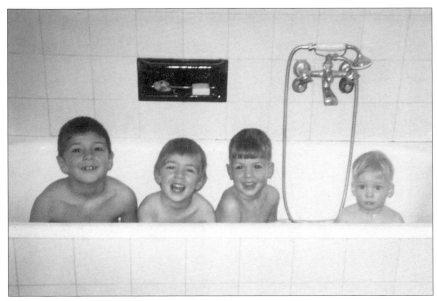

Saturday nights were reserved for bath time with my brothers Paul, John, and Phil.

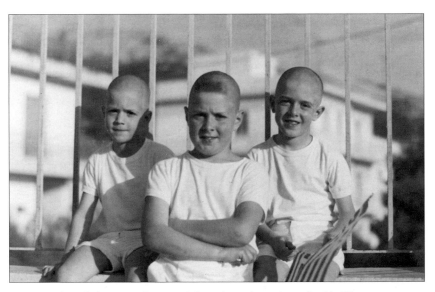

I sported some serious peach fuzz at my elementary school in Athens.

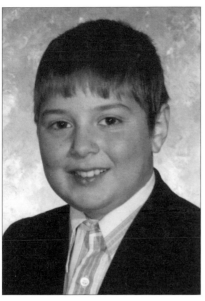

I started becoming pudgy during middle
school in Tenafly, New Jersey.

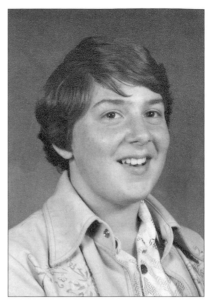

By the time I reached high school,
I felt the pounds creeping up on me.

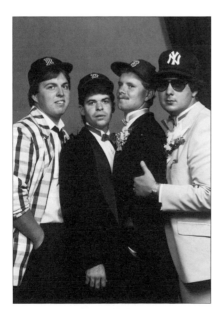

I walked to the beat of my own drum
while attending a formal banquet with
some college buddies.

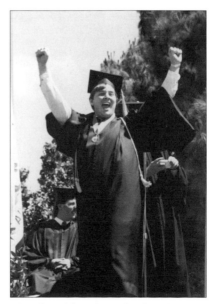

I graduated from Azusa Pacific University
with big hopes for becoming a huge
success in life. Little did I know . . .

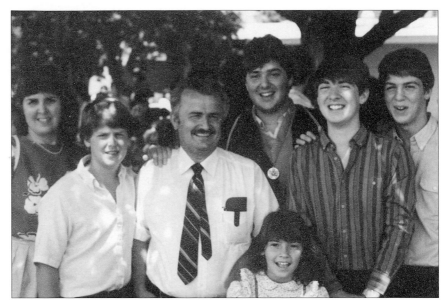

My parents were big on education. They always said,
"It's better to use your head than your hands."

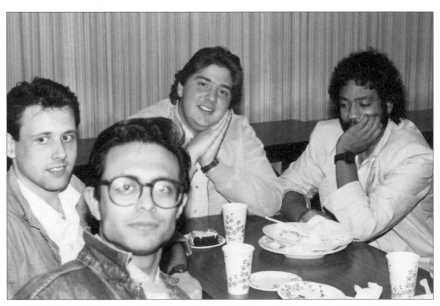

While in graduate school at the age of twenty, I ate and ate—and gained and gained.

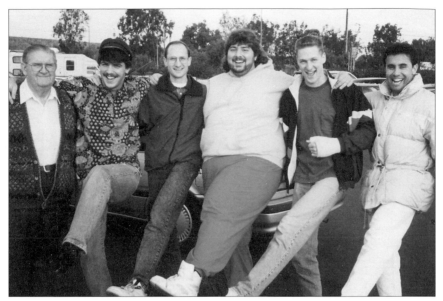

By my mid-twenties, I tried to hide my bloated body behind loose-fitting, baggy clothing.

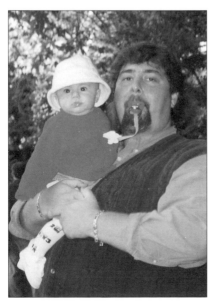

My niece Nicole looked confused when Uncle Nick enjoyed her binky.

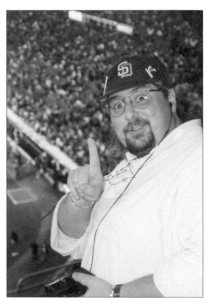

My two favorite teams squared off at the 1998 World Series at Yankee Stadium.

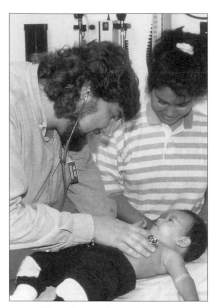

My patients referred to me as
the "big man with the huge heart."

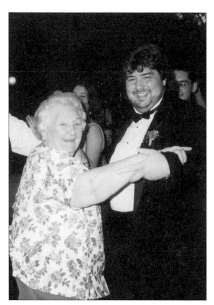

I took over the dance floor with my dear
grandmother Angie Pfaff at my brother
Phil's wedding.

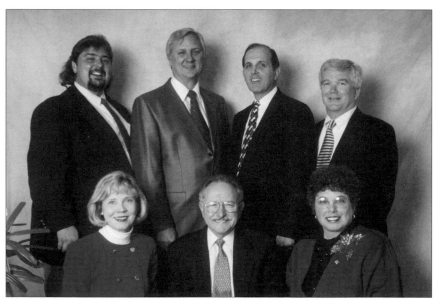

I served as a publicly elected member of the Board of Directors
of the Palomar Pomerado Health System in the late 1990s.

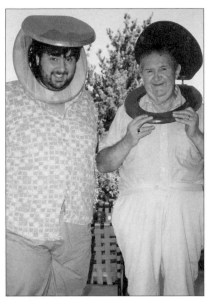

A little bathroom humor with my grandfather
John Pfaff at our Escondido home.

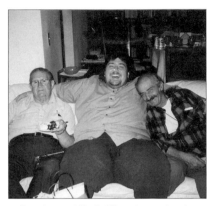

Grandpa and Uncle Elias share a laugh.

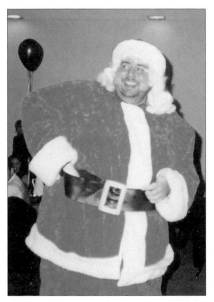

The good thing about being Jolly St. Nick
is that I didn't need any pillows to fill out
my Santa outfit.

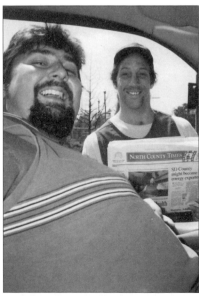

Before the start of my weight-loss tour
in 2001, the local media picked up
on the story.

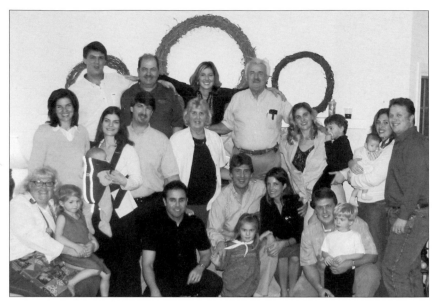

Thanksgiving 2003, a day that I will never forget when I asked Despina to marry me and become part of our big fat Greek family.

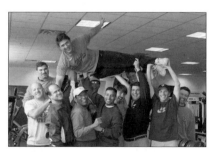

On the day of my bachelor party, my gym-mates celebrated my impending marriage by lifting me into the air. Can you imagine them doing that prior to April Fool's Day 2001?

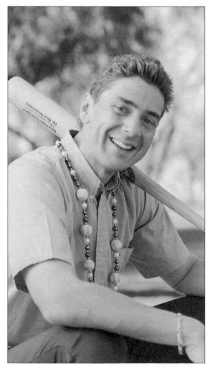

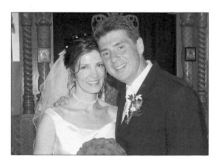

May 1, 2004, the day I married my sweet Despina and gained 120 pounds.

I've loved baseball all my life, so it's appropriate that I took a swing at weight loss. You can hit one out of the park too!

own kitchens. They are folks who live to eat, not eat to live. Do you love food that much? Are you the type who builds your day around food, frequenting the finest restaurants, complimenting the chef before you leave, and telling others what a great meal you enjoyed? It's amazing how people's fascination with food and its preparation have led to a whole plethora of entertaining cooking shows.

For much of my life, I preferred quantity to quality when it came to restaurant meals. I was far happier going back for my fourth plate of pasta at a cheap all-you-can-eat buffet than sampling a fist-sized serving of wild hare roasted with a Barolo sauce and juniper berries. The word *presentation* didn't mean a thing to me. Besides, I couldn't afford $100 dinners as a public health physician serving the uninsured; it just wasn't in the budget.

But when I was elected to the Palomar Pomerado Health Board in 1996, a whole new world opened up to me—the world of *haute cuisine*. Suddenly, people with resources were eager to wine and dine me, and all it took was one look at my massive midsection to understand that the way to my heart was through my stomach. Not that I could be bought for a chateaubriand, but I rather enjoyed feasting on exquisite food on someone else's nickel. Life didn't get better than that. I was invited to special dinners at some of San Diego's finest eateries in the Gaslamp Quarter, La Jolla's Prospect Street, and the seaside restaurants at Del Mar. *I can get used to this,* I said to myself, and I did.

TRAP #4: NURTURE EATING

Do you replace physical intimacy, emotional intimacy, or even sexual intimacy with food? Nurture eating is close to emotional eating, but in this area, food takes on a mystical dimension. Food has the capacity to express love when it's prepared and served in this fashion. We've all seen "Mama Mia" bring out pasta by the kilo and insist that you take a third helping.

Parents continually nurture their children with food. My mother, though she is not from the land of my forefathers, made it a point to learn Greek cooking. She can cook Greek delicacies better than many Greek women I know. When we lived in Greece, she had the reputation of being a Madame of Hospitality. If you happened to drop by my parents' home, within the next ten minutes, Mom would make you feel so comfortable that you would feel like you were in your own home. Nurture eating and nurture feeding can be a positive thing, but nonetheless, it can be overdone.

TRAP #5: CRAVE EATING

Are there certain foods you can't let go of? Certain things you must have? If it's topped with bruschetta, dipped in butter, or covered with chocolate, are you defenseless? It's okay to say yes; I fought food urges most of my adult life. I felt that whenever the craving for a certain food or dessert became too great, I had to give in because the jones wouldn't go away. Crave eating is much like an addiction, and perhaps it needs to be dealt with as such. It's a curiosity to come up with the explanation of why our bodies crave certain things with such intensity. And while it's subjective and variable, certain foods like chocolate elicit yearnings that are hard for science to explain. There's nothing wrong with eating chocolate, but eating a pound of Toblerone is out of control.

TRAP #6: SHAMEFUL EATING

I can confirm that I was a shameful eater. I stuffed more fast-food wrappers and Jack in the Box bags under my car seat than I care to remember, or I furtively tossed them out at work. When I sneaked around with those wrappers, I felt like an IV drug user hiding his syringes or an alcoholic stashing his empties behind a tree. No way my family could see me cleaning out my Expedition at home.

Shameful eaters often pig out in response to guilt or something from the past. They eat out of regret or remorse for personal actions. Some eat to mask pain from childhood trauma, such as being sexually abused by their mother's boyfriend or their brother's friend. Food is often readily available to children, unlike drugs and alcohol, to help them deal with unpleasant feelings.

I have carried on many conversations with women who confessed that after they lost weight, an unexpected thing happened. Some of these women, after being obese for much of their lives, suddenly had male vultures circling them. This attention unfortunately brought back the recollection of inappropriate male attention received early in life. Much to my shock and dismay, numerous women confessed to me that they allowed themselves to regain the weight as a hedge of protection from this leering and preying male attention.

Though I can't relate to their horror stories, I can totally understand them. Medical studies suggest that many victims of abuse end up becoming obese. Nonetheless, I know there are more appropriate ways of dealing with those issues, and I feel that seeking professional psychological and emotional assistance would be absolutely necessary in these cases. A good physician can direct patients to receiving such help when it's needed. Faith-based or employer assistance programs are other options to consider.

It's humbling how food can enter into the equation of some of life's most unexpected challenges. It's yet another example where food is being utilized for a purpose and a role that have no place in our lives.

TRAP #7: BINGE EATING

If the first six traps of eating are the why, then #7—Binge Eating—is the how. Binge eaters go through frequent episodes of compulsive overeating, failing to stop when they're full. Unlike those with bulimia, however, they do not purge their bodies of food. Instead, they feel shame and guilt over this form of self-destructive eating.

Binge eaters are sometimes "hedged hedonists," willing to eat unhealthily but compensate for it afterward. This would be the person who binges on two pints of Starbucks JavaChip ice cream but believes that doing a hundred sit-ups and drinking four cups of water will cancel everything out.

I wasn't a binge eater because I ate around the clock. Binge eaters are more likely to be women who feel shame and remorse for something from their past. They binge on food to forget their pain for a moment. I recommend psychiatric intervention for those fighting this eating disorder, and some require hospitalization.

I like to tell people that in the court of human eating, I plead guilty as charged to the first six counts. I received a lifetime sentence from the judge—467 pounds—until my weight-loss odyssey paroled me from my eating prison.

EATING FOR THE RIGHT REASONS

When I became a cancer survivor, I gave serious thought to what I wanted to do the rest of my life. I understood much, much better how precious a gift life was. Now that I had been given a second chance, what did I want to do with the opportunity?

Lose weight.

Stop being obese.

Live a normal life at an appropriate weight for my height.

So how should I lose weight? I knew that if I ate fewer calories and exercised more, I would shed pounds. I had to. When the formula for losing is distilled to its very essence, it's all about what you put in and what the body exerts. I had relayed that simple formula to my overweight patients for years. Then I went on my eight-month weight-loss journey, and I learned that losing weight is more than eating less and exercising more. I discovered that slashing your calories is all about learning *why* you eat and *how* you eat. Until you take this strategic pillar to heart, you will have great difficulty losing weight and keeping it off.

Why we eat and how we eat are more important than what we eat, but I will be making specific recommendations about the best foods to eat and what to avoid in the next chapter. For now, let me explain why diets don't work. If I outlined a diet plan that dictated, "Don't eat this," or "Do eat that," you'd still be eating for the wrong reasons. Under such a scenario, weight loss and good health would be impossible.

Take myself as an example. I tried the Atkins "revolutionary diet," which limits carbohydrates so that your body can burn fat. The South Beach diet follows a similar low-carb concept. For several weeks, I gorged myself with creams and meats and bacon and cheeses and eggs to the point of almost getting sick. My craving for carbs became so intense, though, that when I fell off the Atkins wagon, I dived into a pound of pasta at Olive Garden and that was that. All the Atkins' dietary restrictions became null and void, and my weight rebounded right back to where it started.

You see, I loved my stomach more than I loved living. I had to stop comforting my stomach and start loving life. The eight-month break from real food was like a detox for me. I learned that food was never intended by God to serve the role it had played in my life.

In essence, I think there is a replacement, a counterfeiting behavior where somehow we allow ourselves to replace the essence of what God intended us to experience with harmful and detrimental behaviors. Tobacco leaves were not placed on the surface of the earth for our smoking pleasure or as an herbal form of Valium. Yet many people claim they smoke because it calms their nerves.

While alcohol may lift the spirits, it was never designed to be the sole coping mechanism with which one can deal with the anguish or pain of past or present personal realities. So, too, food was not designed to be a source of companionship, anxiety relief, or a way of dealing with guilt or shame. While there is nothing wrong with enjoying the experience—and I'm all for eating the highest quality, most delicious food and enjoying it in the process—a healthy balance must be sought. Marc David, author of *Nourishing Wisdom: A Mind-Body Approach to Nutrition and Well-Being,* once said, "Eating is life. Each time we eat, the soul continues its earthly journey. With every morsel of food swallowed, a voice says, 'I choose life.' I choose to eat and I yearn for something more."

GUT-CHECK TIME

In baseball, I love it when the game reaches its climactic moment: bottom of the ninth inning, bases loaded, two out, full count, and the home team down by one run. For every player in the game, it's gut-check time.

It's probably not the bottom of the ninth inning for you, but you're batting with the bases loaded every time you sit down with a plate of food. What are you going to do with that food? Are you going to keep eating and eating, even though, if you did a gut check, you would know that you're full? Here are some other questions to ponder:

- Have you been served more than you should eat?
- Do you have to finish everything on your plate?
- What will you say when you're offered seconds?

Every slender person I know is not skinny because she has been following the Atkins' diet since birth or because she eats more cabbage than anything else. People who have never struggled with their weight—don't you hate them?—eat for the right reason in the right way.

Am I making myself clear here? Losing weight is not about what you eat. It's not about the diet. You have been lied to, and I have been lied to. *The pounds will melt away . . . lose thirty pounds in thirty days . . . a new scientific breakthrough to weight loss.* Diets are a waste of time. Sure, they may work for a season, such as helping you lose twenty pounds to fit into a wedding dress or a tuxedo for an upcoming marriage, but diets miss the whole point. The point is that you need to focus on the way you eat. It's all about the eating behavior—not the content of what goes down the pipe. If you're waiting for me to unveil my secret diet, then you should shut this book right now.

I have this sneaky feeling that you're reading *My Big Fat Greek Diet* because you need to lose a lot more than twenty pounds. You've tried all the diets, just as I have. You've failed every time you resumed your regular lifestyle. Like a cowboy throwing saddlebags on his trusty steed, the pounds came back that fast.

What you need to do is eat for the right reasons in the right way. If it was the food that made you fat, then anyone who ever ate a Twinkie, anyone who ever ate a handful of Oreo cookies, or anyone who ate KFC would be obese. It has nothing to do with the food exclusively. Publishers are churning out how-to diet books by the dozens because overweight people have been convinced that weight loss is one more try away.

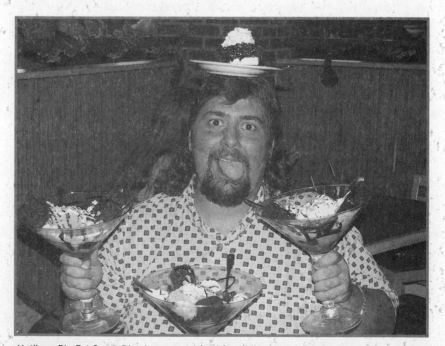

Until my Big Fat Greek Diet, I consumed food for all the wrong reasons.

The irony is that because people are eating for the wrong reasons, they will lose weight the wrong way. Obese people may eat the low-fat version of potato chips, but they'll end up eating twice as much because the low-fat chips taste like flavored cardboard. Their cravings are not satisfied eating the low-fat chips with olestra, a fat substitute that is not absorbed by the intestines and can be very disruptive to your digestive tract. Because olestra isn't absorbed, it just passes through the digestive tract, which can cause significant cramping and diarrhea.

So ultimately, it's like paying a little extra for a flight from San Diego to New York with three layovers versus taking the nonstop flight, paying a little more, and having all that valuable time left over. I would rather take advantage of the best-quality food, but do it in the right way and eat it for the right reasons.

The point that I finally learned is that I had to eat in response to the body's signal of hunger. How to eat to the point of being full is a difficult but simple lesson to learn, and we'll get our hands on this topic in the next chapter.

CHAPTER ELEVEN

PILLAR III:
FILL YOUR TANK WITH THE RIGHT AMOUNT OF THE RIGHT FOODS

I visited dozens and dozens of fast-food restaurants during my weight-loss odyssey across America. Since I always had a traveling companion with me, and he wasn't dieting, we stopped so he could get something to eat. Sometimes we stepped into a fast-food place so I could purchase a diet drink or rendezvous with friends when I was passing through.

Whenever I plopped myself down in a fast-food joint, I sipped a diet soda or a sugar-free iced tea while folks ate their bacon cheeseburgers, chicken deluxe sandwiches, French fries, and onion rings. Early on, I found it difficult to cope with the alluring smells of fried food, but I probably committed the sin of foodography a few times. While everyone was

149

busy munching away and licking their fingers, I would look around the restaurant to give myself something to do. Like the great Yankee catcher Yogi Berra once said, "You can observe a lot by watching."

As a student of human nature, here's what I observed. Not everyone who eats fast food is overweight or obese. I watched people from all walks of life approach the counter and order something to eat, and many looked to be in good shape. Other times when families came into a fast food restaurant, invariably there would be one or two overweight children, or maybe one of the parents was quite heavy.

I watched the way these families ate, and it struck me that those with significant weight issues not only ate all their food, but they scarfed up any stray leftovers on the table. They were the ones devouring every last bite of their hamburgers, "bogarting" someone else's French fries, licking the cheese off the wrapping paper, finishing their kids' half-eaten sandwiches, and returning to the counter for a dessert sundae.

Almost as consistently, I noticed that people *without* a weight problem did not eat all their food. They would slowly chew on two-thirds of their hamburger, three-fourths of their burrito, or two pieces of fried chicken and wrap the leftovers to take home or toss in the trash.

This behavior fascinated me so much that I remember walking up to a middle-aged mother in Kansas. "Excuse me, ma'am," I said with a smile, "but I'm a physician from California, and I noticed that you ate only part of your hamburger and wrapped up the rest. May I kindly ask why you didn't finish your burger?"

"Because I was full," she said.

"How did you know you were full?"

"Because I'm satisfied. I ate enough."

"Don't you feel bad that you paid for it, and you didn't eat it all?"

"Not really."

"But the food tasted good, right?"

"Yeah, but now I'm satisfied."

I must have approached more than a dozen folks during my trip and received similar answers. Those in good shape said they stopped eating because they were satisfied. When their stomachs said that was enough, they stopped eating—no matter how much food was "wasted."

We can learn from that philosophy of eating, and that message underscores my third pillar: Fill your tank with the right amount of the right foods. The "right amount" means learning to stop eating when you're feeling full, and the "right foods" means being selective about what you eat.

This pillar is similar to something Benjamin Franklin said centuries ago: "To lengthen thy life, lessen thy meals."

TRAFFIC LIGHTS AHEAD

If there's one strategic thing I could teach you about eating, it's that the body always sends signals that it's reaching or has reached satiety. The problem is that you've been ignoring those signals for years, perhaps decades. Now those signals are so faint that you'd need a doctor's stethoscope to hear them. Here's how you can recognize those signals and stop eating when you're appropriately full.

I cannot deny that I was tone-deaf when my stomach gently rang a hand bell that said, *Nick, you can stop sending food down here.* I didn't want to hear that because I didn't want to stop eating. I kept chewing and swallowing past the point of appropriate satisfaction. Don't forget I was the type who—after polishing off a twenty-ounce bag of Doritos—reached into the bag and ran my right index finger along the bottom crease, soaking up every last crumb.

That compulsive behavior is the reason I had to learn—the hard way—the following two key concepts. If you can grasp and apply these ideas, I absolutely guarantee that you will lose weight and naturally maintain it. The two points are:

1. **Eat only when you're truly hungry.**
2. **Stop eating when you're appropriately satisfied, not packed.**

We already talked about eating for the right reasons in the last chapter. My question for you now is: When was the last time you really felt hungry? Do you know what hunger pains feel like? Few overweight people do. Just as humorist Will Rogers said he never met a man he didn't like, heavy people never met a meal they didn't like. I never knew what hunger was until April 2, 2001, the second day of my diet. It was a revelation to feel a growing sense of urgency developing in the pit of my stomach, which was starting to grind in my gut. I also felt an ever-so-delicate sense of light-headedness because my blood sugar was dropping steadily.

Hunger is a hard thing to describe to someone who's never experienced it, but it's the kind of thing you should know about because you will be hungry when you lose weight. I doubt many of you have ever experienced true physiological hunger. I'm not talking the munchies here; I'm talking an aspect of the human condition more complicated than that. Until you know what hunger is, you won't be able to stop eating when the body is appropriately satisfied.

When you're trying to lose weight, a delicate balance must be struck between becoming ravenously hungry and allowing the body to develop a slight sense of hunger. These days, I don't allow my hunger to get too out of control because I don't want to go back to those bad old days when I stuffed my face with a bag of Doritos before dinner. To ward off the munchies, I partake of frequent healthy snacks. Midmorning, I will chomp on a juicy red apple. In the afternoon, I'll grab a power bar. After dinner, I'll eat a handful of almonds, along with a diet soda. What I've noticed is that appropriate snacking keeps me from becoming excessively hungry at lunchtime or dinnertime. I mean, I still desire food, but I'm not so famished that I could eat a section of linoleum flooring.

Once you learn how to eat when you're hungry, then you'll learn how to stop eating when you're appropriately satisfied, not packed. When I eat a regular meal, I listen to my body, and when my stomach feels appropriately full, I set my fork and knife on my plate. What does full mean to you? Have you thought about that question lately? Full should be a feeling of all-around satisfaction, a feeling that says, *If I ate another chicken breast, I'd be stuffed.*

Some of us eat beyond the built-in signals of satisfaction. Our stomachs have long ago stopped grinding. The salivary juices are no longer flowing. The light-headed agitation has passed. Yet we forge on and keep shoveling food down our gullets, though a level of discomfort is mounting in our stomachs. Why do people eat and eat when they're beyond full? That's the question of the ages in the weight-loss world.

Several months before I set off on my baseball trip, I woke up on

Thanksgiving morning and found Mom in the kitchen, massaging the turkey with various herbs and spices just before she lifted the bird into the oven. My job—one I volunteered for every year—was to prepare the stuffing, which, in our household, was cooked separately. Regular old cornbread stuffing doesn't cut it in the Yphantides family, so I kicked it up a notch by adding bacon, sausage, pecans, macadamia nuts, dried cranberries, apples, and raisins to the stuffing. On this particular Thanksgiving morning, I sampled the bacon and sausage to make sure it was thoroughly cooked, which is always a good idea when you're serving pork. I sampled several times just to be sure.

I also made extra stuffing batter because a Dr. Nick specialty on Thanksgiving morning was making pancakes from the stuffing mix. A dollop of batter on the grill, and within minutes, I served my family their stuffing pancakes. Those babies, when topped with melted butter and maple syrup, were mighty filling.

After breakfast, I helped Mom prepare the side dishes: mashed potatoes loaded with Parmesan cheese; sweet potatoes covered with marshmallows, brown sugar, and mixed nuts; homemade sourdough rolls; and green beans covered in a creamy dressing and topped with shallot crisps. Chefs have to sample as they cook, right?

By the time the turkey came out of the oven—and my brother John finished deep-frying a second turkey on the back porch—I was already feeling pretty full. I volunteered to carve up the turkeys. Although I wasn't very hungry, I acted like a kid counting garage sale money—one for me, one for you. I think I consumed as much turkey as I put on the serving plates. My father rang the family bell at one o'clock, signaling that our clan could sit down for Thanksgiving dinner.

After Dad said the blessing, we passed around the turkey and all the fixings. I took a generous sampling each time a plate was handed to me, and then I proceeded to stuff myself like a Civil War soldier stuffs a cannon—tight and hard.

Did I save room for dessert? No, but that didn't stop me from feasting on generous wedges of pumpkin pie, German apple pie, and pecan pie topped with whipped cream and French vanilla ice cream. Now I was feeling pain—pain so bad that I ran to the bathroom, where I spontaneously vomited.

That Thanksgiving, I didn't listen to my stomach or pay attention to the dire warning signals my body was sending. I blithely ate my way past the discomfort level, which was a very unhealthy thing to do. It was like I was driving down a four-lane boulevard and cruised right through a red stoplight.

What I did that Thanksgiving—and way too often the other 364 days of the year—was to not pay attention to my body's signals, which are much like traffic signals. A green light means you're hungry, so go ahead and eat. A yellow light is a cautionary reminder that you should stop soon—very soon. A red light means slam on the brakes—now!

Many obese people run a red light every time they sit down with a fork, knife, or spoon in their hands. They're so used to ignoring the body's yellow-light signals that they have no clue what it's like to not eat past the point of appropriate satisfaction.

What about you? Have there been times when you've been full—and a yellow signal is warning you to stop—but you kept on eating because you wanted to? I'm sure that's happened to you. But if you can start paying closer attention to what your body is saying as you eat, you can teach yourself to recognize yellow caution signals. The signs to look for are:

- Your hunger pains are gone.
- You no longer have feelings of light-headedness, low blood sugar level, or mild agitation.
- You have no hunger pains, but your stomach doesn't feel overly full. It feels just right.
- You have a sense of satisfaction and well-being.

If you've been running red lights for years, it's not going to be easy to stop eating when your body sends a blinking yellow-light signal. You're used to keeping the foot on the gas even when your stomach says it's had enough! You can start training your body to brake for yellow lights by asking yourself these questions as you eat:

- "Is my body saying that I've had enough?"
- "Is my stomach satisfied?"
- "Am I full yet?"

If you can truthfully answer yes to any of these questions, you have to walk away from food. I'll let you in on a little secret of the slender world. These questions are second nature to those who weigh less than 150 pounds. Remember the mother in Kansas who didn't finish her fast-food burger? She wrapped up her leftovers because her stomach said she had had enough. What came naturally to her is something that we fatties must learn. We must be aware of how much food we're being served. We must be aware of how much we've eaten.

We must stop eating when we feel full. Not only is it bad for you to continue eating when your stomach is satiated, the food doesn't taste that good. Have you ever noticed during Thanksgiving dinner that all the turkey and trimmings bursting with flavor a half hour ago have lost their appeal? That's because food becomes less tasty the fuller you become. Please keep in mind, however, that it takes a little time for your stomach to send a "Hey, I'm satisfied" signal to your brain. Eating more slowly will give your body time to "get the message" before you have already passed the yellow light.

I have another illustration to drive home the point. The stethoscope has been a cornerstone piece of medical equipment since 1816. When I was taught to use a stethoscope in medical school, I was so preoccupied with using it correctly that I barely paid attention to what I heard in the earpieces. It was months before I could accurately interpret the murmurs of the heart and breath sounds from the lungs.

Fifteen years later, my ears have been trained to listen and interpret the sounds that the body emits when I place the head of the stethoscope on a patient's chest. I can assure you that using my stethoscope has become as natural as tying my shoe. I don't even think about it any more. This is what you should aim for when you're learning to eat the right way. You want to gracefully stop eating and perform a push-up—make that a push-out—from the table. Do this for several weeks, and you will never think of intentionally running a red light again.

YOU'LL GET ENOUGH

I haven't forgotten the sense of urgency I felt when I was around food back in my obese days. I had to eat! Whenever I was invited to a buffet or a party, I approached food as if it were a short-term commodity that would quickly disappear from the face of the earth if I didn't eat it. My parents, who warned me to clean my plate every time we sat down for dinner, had ingrained that feeling in me. I can still hear Mom's admonition ringing in my ears: "Nick, your father worked hard to bring home that food for you."

It took me a long time—try eight months—to realize that food would be available tomorrow. We are blessed to live in a country where supermarkets are as plentiful as spring mushrooms and are filled with aisle after aisle of delicious foodstuffs. This immigrant's son understands that God has blessed Americans with a bounty unprecedented in human history. So what was I worried about all those years? That I wouldn't have enough to eat? That thinking was ludicrous because food is everywhere.

An epiphany came to me during the second week of my weight-loss odyssey. I was attending a Padres game at Qualcomm Stadium when my nostrils detected the smell of garlic fries being eaten in my section. Let me tell you something about garlic fries. There's nothing that could make my gut whistle more than piping-hot garlic fries. Garlic must be in my Greek blood because it's one of my favorite herbal spices. But that evening at the ballpark, I had time to reflect on some things since I wasn't eating. You know what I said to myself? *Nick, the garlic fries will be here next year.* What did I have to worry about? Garlic fries would be available next season at the Gordon Biersch stand inside the ballpark. I didn't need to eat them right then and right now. While I was contemplating this rather profound thought during the Padres game, a series of interconnected thoughts hit me:

- By disciplining myself with the protein shake diet, I would lose weight.

- By losing weight, I would become healthier.
- By becoming healthier, I would live longer.
- By becoming healthier, I would live longer.
- By living longer, I would have more time on this earth to enjoy eating things like garlic fries.

Ding, dong, the wicked witch is dead . . . Wow . . . I could lose weight. Be healthier. Live longer. And have more time to enjoy eating. I mean, *Hello!* I look back on that false sense of urgency—that food would evaporate if I didn't eat it—and realize how ridiculous my thinking was. I told myself, "Stay with the program, bozo. It's all going to work out in the long run."

Lifestyle reprogramming and eating reeducation are tough things to do, which is why losing weight is so difficult. None of us want to change. It's hard. It's painful. But the reason Americans are losing the Battle of the Bulge is because diets don't work. If you approach a diet with a mentality that you're experiencing a temporary deprivation until you return to the way you ate in the past, you're doomed to fail. Trust me. I went that route dozens of times, and I came up empty—or was it full?—every time.

What you have to do is listen to your stomach when it tells you that you've eaten enough—and stop eating.

THE RIGHT FOOD

There's a great scene in the 1973 Woody Allen movie *Sleeper*, in which Allen's character is thawed out after two hundred years in a deep freeze. He wakes up in 2173 a hungry man. The scientists in the room gag, though, when Woody requests a meal of wheat germ, organic honey, and tiger's milk. The thought of eating popular health food, circa 1973, is repulsive to them.

The first scientist informs the other that those were considered healthy foods back then.

"You mean there was no deep fat, no steak or cream pies or hot fudge?" the other scientist exclaimed.

"Those were thought to be unhealthy," the first scientist explained. "Precisely the opposite of what we now know to be true."

I have to laugh when I hear that story because it seems that every year we hear about the latest food fad or food diet. From choking on bacon with Atkins, to eating with a calculator with Zone, to having sand in your food with South Beach, to tracking points with Weight Watchers, the weight-loss world is eager to tell you what to eat.

For a price, of course. Sometimes it's the cost of a book; other times it's buying their specially produced MREs—meals ready to eat. While most diet books have merit, it's a bald-faced lie to say that food selection is the key to optimal health. LOSING WEIGHT IS NOT ABOUT THE FOOD. Eliminating certain foods or constantly depriving yourself of something you enjoy will cause more harm than good. So I say, pick a diet. Any diet. Just do it and stick with it. But don't pick one that's going to test your willpower when it denies certain foods to you. As author Rick Warren said, "Most diets don't work because they keep you thinking about food all the time, guaranteeing you'll be hungry."

Now, I can tell that my advice isn't enough for you. I know what you're thinking: *Dr. Nick, you can't leave me hanging like this. You've got to tell me how to eat the right way. You've got to tell me what to eat.*

Okay, I'm game. I'll tell you what I eat—and how I eat. I follow a modified Atkins' diet. I limit certain carbohydrates and sugars but not selectively or militantly. Limiting carbohydrates is a guideline, not an absolute. Thus, I stay away from sandwiches, pastas, rice, and potatoes because they have a high glycemic index. The glycemic index is a ranking of foods based on their immediate effect on blood sugar levels. It is a measure of how quickly the carbohydrates in a food are broken down into simple sugars. Carbohydrate foods with a high glycemic index—white breads, starchy potatoes, and sugary desserts—raise your blood sugar levels dramatically and rapidly. When blood sugar levels are high, cells tend to burn sugar more than they burn fat, reducing the amount of fat burned in your body.

Naturally, it's better to eat foods with a low glycemic index. This would be certain fruits, vegetables, salads, and whole wheat products. A book I enjoyed, *Sugarbusters*, provides a very detailed summary on this issue. I also eat plenty of protein contained in meat. Because of my weight training, I have increased my protein intake by consuming large amounts of chicken, seafood, pork, and beef.

A typical breakfast for me is a bowl of warm oatmeal or whole grain cereal with skim milk. I used to be a Lucky-Charms-or-Coco-Puffs-drenched-in-whole-milk type of guy, but now I'm pleased with cereals like Kashi Go-Lean Crunch or Quaker Oats bran. I've ditched the whole milk and substituted skim milk or soymilk.

Midmorning, I fortify myself with an apple, pear, or orange. Sometimes I'll have some cottage cheese with figs or persimmons.

For lunch, I make myself an adventurous salad, but I use a limited amount of dressing. I don't necessarily use a low- or nonfat salad dressing either, but I forgo the croutons. For an afternoon snack if I'm hungry, I'll eat a power bar like the Zone fudge graham bar or the peanut butter caramel bar.

For dinner, I like to see a good piece of fish or grilled chicken on my plate surrounded by a generous helping of broccoli, asparagus, or green beans. I usually have a small salad as well, but I'm light on the dressing.

For dessert, I'll eat a handful of raw almonds or dried fruit. Once in a great while, I will enjoy a not-so-healthy sweet like a warm chocolate chip cookie, but no more than one or two at a time.

You're probably wondering what I eat in restaurants, which is a great question. These days, I'll order a small house salad as an appetizer *and* a dinner salad as my entrée, such as a Cobb salad, holding the eggs, or a Greek salad with extra feta cheese. I always request that my dressing arrive separately on the side. If I happen to order a regular meal, I'll substitute the starch carbohydrate (baked potato or rice) with extra vegetables or cottage cheese.

If I returned to Ruth's Chris Steak House, it wouldn't resemble the all-out food orgy I experienced during the Last Supper. I would skip the appetizers, and instead of the forty-ounce porterhouse steak for two, I would order the more modest rib eye steak, weighing in at sixteen ounces. I would tell the waiter not to bring any potato sides to the table, but I would treat myself to one piece of bread. If I had any takers, I would share one dessert with those joining me for the meal.

I'm not a maniac about what I eat. I've maintained my weight for three years by eating like a normal person, not like an obese person. While I avoid certain kinds of food, I haven't eliminated everything. I confess that I've eaten French fries. I even treated myself to a serving of garlic fries at the Padres' Opening Day in 2002. Just as I predicted, the Gordon Biersch stand still sold them.

What you eat is all about listening to your body, moderating your serving sizes, and stopping when you're full. These concepts can be summed up in this way:

DR. NICK'S TEN COMMANDMENTS
OF HEALTHY EATING

1. Stop eating when your body gives you the yellow caution signal.

While we should delight in the wonders of food, we must remember that at the end of the day, we're eating to satisfy our hunger. This means we must stop eating when our body has reached a point of appropriate satisfaction.

2. Avoid food wrapped in plastic, sealed in a can, or not served in its original form.

The majority of foods wrapped in plastic contain large quantities of processed sugar, processed flour, and saturated fats. This, of course, is to satisfy the sweet tooth and the fat stomachs of Americans. I avoid food products stripped of their nutrient values through excessive processing. You can bet your bottom dollar that anything baked outside your home includes white processed flour, which has a high glycemic index.

One of the best things to happen to me after I resumed eating solid food was that I could eat *only* vegetables. Back in my bad old days, I sneered at asparagus or cauliflower on my plate. I viewed them as decorative items, something akin to a floral centerpiece. Since I had disdained vegetables before Thanksgiving 2001, I couldn't see how I could build my diet around plain old green beans and mushrooms.

That mind-set changed when my taste buds were reintroduced to vegetables between Thanksgiving and Christmas. They tasted wonderful! These morsels of deliciousness, bursting with flavor, wowed even my jaded palate. It's exciting to kick up veggies a notch with a variety of spices and herbs. After that, vegetables—along with fruits and nuts—became the cornerstone of my diet.

3. Limit your processed carbohydrates and increase your intake of complex carbohydrates.

I was a grab-and-go guy during my obese days—grab a chocolate éclair at the 7-Eleven after a fill-up, go for the blueberry muffins in the break room or the bagel smeared with cream cheese at the office birthday party.

Those food items are distant memories. I'm not saying that I haven't taken a bite of a processed sweet, but now I try to eat foods with a low glycemic index like whole grain and whole wheat breads, wild rice, cracked wheat, whole wheat pasta, and an assortment of whole grain crackers and crispy bread.

If you crave bread, then you should buy a bread machine and make bread with unprocessed wheat flour purchased in bulk from a health food store.

4. Fill the hunger hole in your stomach with salads and other healthy options before you plow into carbohydrates and fats.

Salads have become my friend, and I've told you how much I enjoy vegetables. If you had told me five years ago that broccoli dusted with Parmesan cheese would be the height of culinary delight for me, I would have ordered psychiatric testing for you.

My taste buds were never like that. In the past, I would inhale a large stuffed-crust pizza or a huge carne asada burrito to satisfy my hunger pains. In a nutshell, I ate sinful food when I was hungry. Bad mistake.

When you're hungry, you're less selective about what you eat because you'll eat anything, even if you *know* it's junk. Why else do the food vendors at the state fair rake in so many bucks selling corn dogs and funnel cakes? Be smart and choose nutritious things to eat, especially when you're hungry. Then even a plain garden salad would be yummy for your tummy.

5. Eat treats like they are treats.

I am not supportive of completely eliminating certain things from your diet as many diet plans suggest. When I deprived myself of something I really wanted, I would subconsciously compensate for that deprivation by excessively eating other alternatives.

For instance, if I saw Mom bring out a homemade Greek custard called *galaktobouriko*, I would try to tell myself, *No, don't eat a piece,* but then I would end up grabbing *five* pieces of baklava an hour later. But if I'd eaten a modest sliver of *galaktobouriko,* that would have been all I wanted.

It's better to eat a modest portion to satisfy the craving than deprive yourself and go crazy later on.

6. Don't waste calories.

This commandment is fundamental to weight-loss maintenance, but it's fairly radical. I've decided that I shall drink nothing with calories. That means no lemonade, no nondiet sodas, and no wine.

My rationale is that I prefer to *eat* my calories. In other words, I would rather have a piece of cheese than a glass of milk. I would rather peel and eat an orange than drink a glass of orange juice. I would rather artificially sweeten my tea than drink "sweet tea," which has so much sugar in it you'd have a heart attack if you saw how it's made. The same goes for diet drinks versus regular sodas.

This personal directive also extends to alcohol. I am convinced that alcohol in moderation, especially red wine, has some health benefits. I've even told Dad that he should drink a few ounces of red wine daily. As for myself, I've never had a problem with alcohol. I used to consume it in healthy moderation, but I haven't sipped any alcohol since the Last Supper. Given the choice between 110 calories in a small glass of wine versus 127 calories in a biscotti, there's no doubt which of the two provides me with greater pleasure these days. So I'm a teetotaler.

Since I no longer drink calories because I want to save my calories for real food, I consume *lots* of water. During the day, I try to drink several glasses of water because not only is it calorie-free, but water's great for the body. In addition, I enjoy lightly sweetened sparkling waters, diet sodas, and artificially sweetened iced tea. The only time I consume any milk is when I eat cereal. I have eliminated thousands and thousands of calories each month by sticking with this guideline, and you can, too, if you choose not to drink anything with calories in it. Sure, it will take a few months to get used to switching over to the "blander" water, teas, and diet sodas, but you're going to be much better off.

There are other ways to "save" on calories in addition to cutting back on sugary soft drinks. You should take an inventory of your eating habits and see where you could painlessly eliminate calories. This would be like cutting the fat from your family budget.

7. Eat tasty and satisfying food.

If you had asked me five years ago if I loved good food, I would have been all over that question. "Nobody loves good food more than me," I would have said, patting my sixty-inch waist to illustrate tangible proof of that statement.

Back then, I thought three-star chefs found in the *Michelin Guide* had nothing over the Colonel, and nobody cooked Italian like Chef Boyardee. But as I moved away from processed food and began to eat more raw fruits and cooked vegetables, my taste buds changed. Fast food, cheap food, ill-prepared food, or canned food no longer tastes as good to me. Put another way: All-you-can-eat buffets and smorgasbords no longer get my business, unless it's a salad buffet with lots of fresh vegetables and succulent fruit.

What gets my mouth watering these days is what some people call the Mediterranean diet, which is built around seafood, olive oil, feta cheese, nuts, and vegetables—nutritious food prepared with thoughtful and deliberate care. These days I'm more careful with what I put into my body, because I want every calorie to count. There's nothing more pleasurable than eating something prepared with love.

8. Kick-start your metabolism every morning.

I never start the day without eating, which is totally the opposite of what I used to do. Don't forget that when I was obese, I officially started my new diet every morning at 7:30, which involved not eating food. (Isn't that about the dumbest thing you've ever heard?) I fasted all morning, and sometimes I managed to skip lunch, but by 2 p.m., the Dr. Jekyll of controlled eating turned into the Mr. Hyde of ravaging consumption. Nobody, and I mean nobody, out-ate me from late afternoon to midnight. If you are actively exercising, a healthy late-night snack is actually okay. Late-night engorgement is not.

The irony is that I would eat right up until I went to bed, retiring with a full belly. As you would expect, I would wake up in the morning still feeling satiated, which prompted thoughts of going on a "diet" again. So I resolved myself to be "good," but once my stomach growled like a pack of wolverines six or seven hours later, Mr. Hyde magically reappeared, and the cycle repeated itself.

I never understood the importance of eating breakfast until I began eating solid food again, which is a sad excuse for a family physician to make, but it's true. If I had eaten a regular breakfast, I could have broken the cycle and given myself a decent shot at making a diet work, but I never had a chance.

The benefits of eating breakfast are well known. Your metabolism—which resembles a furnace—doesn't get fired up until it's stoked with fuel. If you don't eat breakfast, the body turns to its own muscle mass—not fat cells!—for energy. As the metabolism slows to a crawl, the body conserves energy because it doesn't know when it's going to receive fuel again. When food is finally eaten at lunchtime or in the afternoon, the body doesn't burn the food for energy but stores it as fat. As you can see, by starving myself each morning, I was doing the exact opposite of what I should have been doing.

It's better to give the body some breakfast each morning, which stokes that furnace and starts burning calories.

9. Keep your body hydrated with plenty of fluids.

Most Americans go through life dehydrated. I see it in my practice every day—kidney stones, dry skin conditions, digestive problems, and an assortment of ailments either directly or indirectly related to inadequate hydration. Many Americans don't even come close to drinking enough water, relying on caffeinated beverages like coffee, sodas, and teas as their exclusive source of liquid intake. There is nothing wrong with some caffeine in and of itself, but exclusively relying on caffeinated beverages for hydration will get you behind in the count faster than you can say Randy Johnson.

Caffeine, which promotes irritability, anxiety, and mood swings, has a diuretic effect that stimulates the kidneys to secrete excess liquids. With time and continued stimulation, the body slowly gets into a water-deprived state, which can compound the various conditions previously discussed. The answer is simple: Drink more water.

Your body needs water in a big way. Water makes up 92 percent of your blood plasma, 80 percent of your muscle mass, 60 percent of your red blood cells, and 50 percent of everything else in your body.

Additionally, there is a practical motivation to increasing water and noncaloric fluid intake. Multiple studies and personal experience have shown that increasing water intake can actually have an appetite-suppressing effect. Taking a big gulp of water mitigates hunger pains and gives you a temporary sense of fullness that can be used advantageously in helping you limit your caloric intake.

I've gone overboard on this concept of drinking water, which is an apt description. I drink so much water that some of my friends have suggested that I apply for a job as a fountain in front of Caesar's Palace in Las Vegas. Ten, fifteen times a day I see visible evidence that I'm drinking more water than in the past. My urine tends to be clear now, compared to the glow-in-the-dark concentrated urine that I used to see in the toilet bowl. Urine that is bright yellow is too concentrated and a sign that the body is not adequately hydrated.

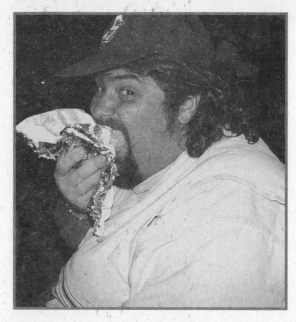

I never entered a hot dog eating contest, but I coulda been a contender. Now I eat much more sensibly. In the old days, I would have eaten half of this roast lamb during our traditional Greek Easter feast, but no longer.

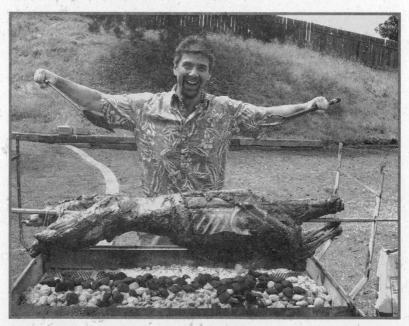

10. Eat frequently to avoid ravaging hunger.

Since I started eating fruit and power bars between meals to "hold" me over to lunch or dinner, I'm able to sit down and consume a more appropriate amount of food than I would if my blood sugar levels were low.

Whenever I was light-headed from skipping meals or from inappropriate snacks, it compromised my judgment of what I should and should not eat. I've learned to consume handfuls of nuts, pieces of fruit, healthy power bars, a piece of cheese, or rolled-up slices of turkey two or three times a day. In Greek, we call it *mezethaki*, which means a little morsel of food can take the edge off hunger. This allows me to then approach the dinner table with better judgment and a more sober-minded temperament.

Now I consume food at the right time in the right way for the right reasons. I feel better, have more energy from the time I wake until I go to bed, and go through the day with a spring in my step. The best thing about following this pillar is that I'll never have to diet again, and neither will you if you follow the principles I've outlined.

CHAPTER TWELVE

PILLAR IV: BURN CALORIES LIKE NEVER BEFORE

While driving through the heartland of America during my weight-loss adventure, an Iowa Highway Patrol officer pulled up next to me with flashing lights. I glanced to my left and saw him jab his finger in the air—the universal gesture to pull over. I immediately slowed down and came to a stop on the interstate shoulder. I assumed I was being stopped for speeding.

"Good afternoon, sir. What did I do wrong?" I asked cheerfully.

"License and registration, please."

"Was I speeding?"

"Proof of insurance please."

Apparently I wasn't going to sweet-talk one of Iowa's finest out of a speeding ticket. I fumbled in the glove compartment for the necessary documents. "But what did I do wrong?" I asked.

This time he ignored me while he studied my driver's license.

Riding in the van with me was Pat Kenney, pastor of my home church in Escondido. I looked over and saw him hastily thumbing through his wallet. "It's got to be here somewhere," he said.

"What?"

"My Escondido PD badge for chaplains."

Hurry. We don't have much time to talk our way out of this one.

The Iowa highway patrolman finally answered my question. "I noticed you're not wearing your seat belt."

I looked down at my massive girth. He was right. My face turned beet red, and shame washed over me. "But sir, it doesn't fit," I said in way of explanation. (This incident happened in late July when I was in the 350-pound range.)

"Where's your medical excuse?"

"You're looking at it," I fired back.

"What do you mean?"

"I'm a medical doctor."

"You're a medical doctor who's so big that you can't get a seat belt around you? Get out of the car."

"Get out of the car?"

"You heard me."

Suddenly, this was turning serious. Was I going to be handcuffed, or worse—be taken in and strip-searched?

The patrolman jerked his head and led me to his vehicle, where he opened the back door to his patrol car. I gulped and got in—barely fitting onto the rear bench seat. Then he closed the door and walked back to the van, where he spent several minutes questioning Pastor Pat about who we were and what we were doing.

When he returned to his squad car, he asked me the same questions to see whether our stories matched. After corroborating our answers, he took out a pad and asked me for my name, address, and phone number, and I steeled myself for an expensive summons. With a grin on his face, he handed me a warning. "You guys are unbelievable. Now get out of Iowa," he said playfully.

If only I had exercised more in life, embarrassing situations like that could have been avoided. I paid dearly for decades of sedentary living. If the reality show *Survivor* were looking for a cast of couch potatoes, my demo video would have landed me a spot on the island. I would have loved showing the producers my idea of exercise: the heavy lifting I did with a fork; the stretches I performed while reaching for a sack of fast food at the drive-thru window; and the deep knee bends I performed when I sat on the throne.

Prior to stepping on a treadmill in San Francisco, I was among the 25 percent of the American population who don't exercise at all, according to the Centers for Disease Control. If you had asked me why back then, I would have replied, "I don't have time to exercise." That's the excuse *du jour* for everyone, isn't it? *I don't have time.* We get up in the morning, go to work, come home, eat dinner, tuck the kids in bed, watch some TV, and go to bed. American society is packed with fat rats running around collecting large piles of cheese that many of them will never have the opportunity to eat. These men and women are chasing success and financial security by devoting their waking hours to getting ahead in the rat race. Others are paddling as fast as they can just to keep the bills paid or avoid falling further into debt. Something has to give, so they sacrifice their physical health on the altar of the Almighty Dollar. But sooner or later, they will pay for their short-sightedness: They will be crippled or die prematurely from disease, or they will have to give up their hard-won financial gain to pay for their deteriorating physical health.

Today, I'm convinced that we don't have time not to exercise. It's become that important. Exercise has become as much a part of my daily routine as brushing my teeth or checking my e-mail. It's my grace zone. Because I exercise, I get to enjoy food again.

If I had not added an exercise component to my lifestyle change, I would be back right where I started on April Fools' Day in 2001. Here's why. These days I vigorously exercise seven days a week for a minimum of one hour, but closer to two hours, each day. I burn an average of 1,000 calories with each workout at my local YMCA. That works out to 7,000 calories per week.

Each pound of human fat is the equivalent of 3,500 calories of stored energy. Were I to continue eating the same amount that I currently am without exercising, I would gain two pounds per week. (That's 7,000 calories I'm burning in the gym divided by 3,500 calories per pound of human fat.) If I gained two pounds a week for fifty-two weeks, that would come to 104 pounds per year. From the time I reached my goal weight in April 2002 to the release of this book in the fall of 2004 (130 weeks), I would regain 260 of the 270 pounds that I lost.

That's scary.

But stay with me here. I know I'm throwing a lot of numbers at you, but consider this. It's a fact that males, to maintain their current weight, consume a baseline of approximately 12 calories for every pound they weigh. (For women, it's 10 calories per pound.) Since I weigh 210 pounds, I multiply 210 times twelve, which gives me a sum of 2,520 calories per day. If I *didn't* exercise, I'd have to limit my eating to 2,520 calories a day if I wanted to remain at 210 pounds. Since I'm burning 1,000 calories a day in the gym, however, I'm able to eat up to 3,500 calories a day and maintain my current weight.

At 3,500 calories per day, I can enjoy complete meals—no "rabbit food" on my plate—with my family. I can have my cake and eat it, too.

Now, I understand the amount of exercise that I am currently doing—one to two hours a day—is drastic. Most busy moms and dads would never have the privilege of spending this much time working out each day. Anyone who has 270 pounds to lose, however, has to make the time, and they have no other choice. (Actually, anyone who has more than fifty pounds to lose will have to make sacrifices and significant schedule adjustments to exercise appropriately.)

The one question I am asked most often when sharing my story in public is, "Dr. Nick—what about the loose skin?" Having lost as much weight as I did, exercise serves an important role as I sculpt my body and reshape my physical image. Let me tell you, however, that the one company I will never represent is Speedo swimwear. I do have an impressive amount of redundant skin, but fortunately, you can't even tell when I'm fully clothed.

Many people who haven't lost even as much weight as I have undergo plastic surgery to remove the sagging folds. The gym is where I am having my "natural" plastic surgery. As I faithfully exercise and build muscle mass, the contour of my body is tightening and my loose skin is slowly receding. I have already seen impressive progress. Call me vain, but when I go swimming at the beaches here in San Diego, I don't want to look like a freak of nature.

Final point: I am not suggesting that anyone who needs to lose weight must work out for one to two hours each and every day. I am suggesting, though, that anyone who has more than a few pounds to lose should make an exercise investment consistent with their goals for weight loss.

NO PAIN, LOTS OF GAIN

Every now and then, I catch an infomercial touting effortless weight loss. I love the one showing the cute, tanned blonde with a black pad of electrodes wrapped around her stomach. Seated languorously in a La-Z-Boy, she struggles to keep her eyes open as the passive electrical stimulation "burns" fat cells and "builds" muscles.

These infomercials burn me up because they're selling a way to lose weight without exercise. Weight loss doesn't work that way! Once you embark on your weight-loss journey, you will *have* to burn calories like never before. That's why the exercise pillar is so important. Weight reduction and maintenance will be impossible to sustain without vigorous physical exertion *for the rest of your life.*

People are duped into buying "fat burners" every day. I've had patients ask me in all seriousness whether they work. With a friendly grin on my face, I tell them that these electrical pads can't work because exercise must stimulate and strengthen the most important muscle in the body—the heart.

The human heart is a miraculous muscle with an electrical network and an incredible adaptability to modify its performance in response to whatever activity you are doing. From sleeping to sitting to walking to running for your life, your heart responds by contracting and forcing your blood, which contains life-essential oxygen and nutrients, into every cell in your body. The cardiovascular system— consisting of the heart, arteries, capillaries, and veins—is the tree trunk of life.

I will never forget during my medical school days when I had the privilege of participating in the first combined heart-lung transplant ever performed at the UCSD Medical Center. I assisted the lead surgeon as he cracked open the patient's chest—a woman in her twenties with a rare heart-lung disease—and removed the entire contents of her thoracic cavity. I was awestruck by the procedure. For the first time, I saw with my own eyes the heart's central location physically and its central role physiologically.

The woman's heart was diseased, flabby, loose, discolored, and scarred. She was a slender woman who suffered from a metabolic disease that affected her heart and lungs. Her only hope of living was a heart-lung transplant.

I helped crack open the chest and used my fingers to hold back soft tissue—sort of a human retractor. My job was to get things out of the way so the lead surgeon would have room to get down deep into the body's cavities.

The transplant heart was a perfectly shaped, brilliant pink, vibrant muscle. To see something so perfectly designed, so perfectly nestled into such a strategic part in the human body, was a reminder to me of what an incredible muscle the heart really is.

Exercise strengthens your ultimate muscle. Your ultimate muscle enables you to keep living. As you exercise and get into shape, you preserve and protect the quality of the heart's blood vessels and prevent heart attacks. The last time I checked, God was giving us only one heart; regular, consistent exercise will help you live longer and keep pounds off. It is with some urgency that I implore you to exercise. Most Americans are not even close to meeting basic activity level recommendations. That's crazy! We have to get people moving.

MAKING THOSE FIRST STEPS

You can choose from any number of sports or physical activities to get in shape and stay in shape. But if you're as obese as I was, you probably haven't been very active, so the thought of playing tennis, signing up for the church softball team, or joining a "spinning" class seems as far-fetched as wearing a bathing suit on a local beach.

Here's my advice: *Get thee to a gym.*

This is nonnegotiable. I will give you a doctor's excuse only if you live in a rural part of the country where gyms are many miles away in the "big city." But if a fitness center is conveniently located near you, then you should join one. Even if you have to max out your credit card to purchase a membership, you should do it. That's how important exercise is. To paraphrase the wit and wisdom of Yankee catcher Yogi Berra, exercise "is 90 percent mental. The other half is physical."

You may be saying, "But Dr. Nick, how do I start?"

Just as I did—with walking on a treadmill (at home or in a gym) or even walking around the neighborhood. Walking places a gentle strain on all parts of the body while gradually imposing mild stress on the heart. That's important when you're starting because you need to build up the heart muscle as you build up stamina.

Walking is a surprisingly effective strategy for weight loss. Don't give me the excuse that you don't have time. Make the time—even if you start with fifteen minutes a day. The idea is to make a commitment to start exercising regularly. By "regularly," I mean doing something physically exerting every single day. If that sounds impossible, may I remind you that if this formerly fat Greek fool could do it, so can you. Daily exercise will take every drop of resolve flowing through your body because fitness is all about patience and perseverance, energy and enthusiasm, and sacrifices and spontaneity. Whether exercise becomes part of your lifestyle will make or break your ability to lose weight and keep it off.

I can hear the excuses coming, but I've heard them all because I've *said* them all. Here's what I have to say to people looking for a loophole not to exercise:

"Dr. Nick, I don't have time in the morning."

Yes, you do. Just wake up earlier. That may mean you have to go to bed earlier, but that's not going to kill you. Most gyms are open by 6 a.m. The best reason for exercising in the morning is that you can't cancel a workout that's already happened. But you have to do what works for you. If you're a morning person, take advantage of that aptitude and get into the gym before you start your day. If noontime at the company gym works best for your schedule, then go with that. If you're a night owl who gets a second wind after dinner, then exercise at night. I exercise at all hours of the day because I have a different schedule every day. It's doesn't matter when you exercise, it just matters that you do.

"Dr. Nick, I don't have time after work."

But you have time after preparing and serving dinner to your family. You can go to the gym or walk around the neighborhood. Ride a bike to a nearby park or swim at a municipal pool. Volunteer at the local humane society and offer to walk their dogs. Isn't your health more important than watching *Entertainment Tonight*?

"But Dr. Nick, there's something good on TV."

You can tape the show for viewing later. You know how to program a DVD or VCR player, don't you? I personally limit my TV watching to news and sports. I'd rather live a sitcom or a captivating reality show than watch one.

"Dr. Nick, I can't get a babysitter."

Most fitness centers offer some sort of child-care arrangement. You can also offer to watch your friend's children in exchange for watching yours while you exercise.

"Dr. Nick, I'm too fat."

All the more reason to exercise. Do you know a better way to lose weight?

"Dr. Nick, I can't afford a fitness center."

You can find gyms in all price ranges. Ritzy, high-end gyms charge $500 and up for initiation, plus $75 to $100 a month in dues. Mid-tier fitness clubs charge $250 and up for initiation and $50 a month for dues. But no-frills clubs located in strip malls often waive their modest $100 or less initiation fees just to get you in the door paying between $25 and $50 a month. Finally, may I make a plug for YMCAs around the country? (Full disclosure: I'm the poster boy for the Palomar

Family YMCA, which has been advertising in newspapers using before-and-after photos of yours truly.) My local Y, which has all the machines and treadmills, costs $34 a month after a $50 initiation fee. YMCAs around the country have similar modest fees.

"Dr. Nick, I don't feel comfortable walking in my neighborhood."

Then find one or two friends who can walk with you. Carry a stick or an old golf club to ward off dogs. Walk during the daylight hours.

"But it's too cold outside."

Well, you can put a stationary bike in front of your television. Another great idea, no matter what part of the country you live in, is to "power walk" in malls. They are great places to exercise because of the temperature-controlled environment and engaging window displays to distract you. However, a leisurely stroll to the food court to get a large order of chili cheese fries does not count!

"I'm a stay-at-home mom with kids."

Purchase a treadmill and walk during naptime or while your husband watches the children. You can also pay a teenager a few dollars to watch your children while you work out.

"Dr. Nick, it hurts my knees to walk on a treadmill."

Then ride a recumbent bike or swim. When your knees get used to physical activity after years without use, you can try walking on a treadmill again.

"But Dr. Nick, you don't know what it's like to be the fattest person in the gym."

Ah, I caught you. Yes, I do know what it's like. But excuses are excuses, and the mind has an amazing ability to rationalize and create excuses to get you out of things you don't want to do. My advice is that when an excuse comes to mind, you immediately think of something else. Your life may depend on it.

BURN CALORIES BY THE BUSHEL

I walked for more than five months before I felt I had enough stamina and confidence to try jogging on the treadmill. As your stamina builds, you can rev up your heart with other types of aerobic exercise—stationary bikes, stair-steppers, cross-country ski trainers, rowing machines, and the newfangled elliptical exercisers, which are a cross between a stationary bike, a cross-country ski machine, and a bit of a stair-climber. They stimulate walking, stepping, and cycling with an elliptical motion as you work your arms, getting a total-body workout.

The idea behind these exercise machines is to burn calories by the bushel. Aerobic exercise is at a pace that allows muscles to use the oxygen that is available to them. What I love about the newer machines is that they come with a computer chip that monitors your heart rate, calories burned, how far you've traveled (or stairs you've climbed), and how long you've been working out.

Since the goal is to burn calories by the bushel, you should be aware that certain machines and certain physical activities take more energy to do. In the gym, this is what a 200-pound person can expect to expend for one hour of exercise:

- Jogging at an eight-minute-per-mile pace: 1,200 calories per hour
- Vigorous stationary bike riding: 1,008 calories per hour
- Jogging at a ten-minute-per-mile pace: 960 calories per hour
- Elliptical trainer general workout: 864 calories per hour
- Jogging at a twelve-minute-per-mile pace: 768 calories per hour
- Moderate stationary bike riding: 672 calories per hour
- Stair-step machine general workout: 576 calories per hour
- Vigorous weight lifting: 576 calories per hour
- Walking at a fifteen-minute-per-mile pace: 432 calories per hour
- General weight lifting: 288 calories per hour

As you can see, jogging on a treadmill gives you the most bang for your exercise buck, but telling overweight and obese people to start running is like telling a pig to fly. It's not going to happen. When I put one foot in front of another at that San Francisco YMCA, that's all I was capable of physically doing—putting one foot in front of the other.

So accept that you'll start with walking, whether it be on a treadmill or outside before you can move up to elliptical trainers, stair-steppers, and riding a stationary bike. That's not only fine, that's great! The important thing is to get the body used to exerting itself after years of inactivity.

When performing aerobic exercise, you need to be aware of your maximum heart rate and your target heart rates. The goal is to raise your heart rate into the "target zone," meaning between 65 percent and 80 percent of your maximum heart rate. I've been pushing myself and trying to get my heart rate up to 160 beats per minute, which is 85 to 90 percent of my maximum heart rate. I know that's a little high, but I've slowly built up to this level.

Check out the Heart Rate Guide below and eyeball what your target heart rate should be. For a more precise formula based on whether you are a beginner or an intermediate exerciser, check out my Web site at healthsteward.com.

TARGET HEART RATE ZONES (IN BEATS/MIN.)

Age	Healthy Heart 50 to 65 percent	Aerobic Training 65 to 80 percent	Predicted Maximum Rate (100 percent)
20	100–130	130–160	200
25	98–127	127–156	195
30	95–124	124–152	190
35	93–120	120–148	185
40	90–117	117–144	180
45	88–114	114–140	175
50	85–111	111–136	170
55	83–107	107–132	165
60	80–104	104–128	160
65	78–101	101–124	155
70	75–98	98–120	150

After you've built up some stamina, I must emphasize that exercise should be painful. Well, not painful as in hurting yourself, but you should exert yourself to the point of gasping for air and producing rivulets of sweat on your forehead. At least some discomfort is the goal here. I start off my daily exercise regimen at the Palomar Family YMCA with thirty to sixty minutes—sixty is more typical—of aerobic exercise on a cross-trainer, treadmill, stair-stepper, or stationary bike. When I'm done, I'm panting like a golden retriever in August, and my workout clothes are soaked from head to toe with drenching sweat. I've been more careful to wipe up after myself after one lady waved her finger in my face and said, "This is disgusting. You're a doctor. You should know better. I don't want to get sick from your sweat."

So I spend extra time wiping up my pools of perspiration. I'm relaying this story to make the point that when I hop on these machines, I'm not out for a Sunday-go-to-meeting stroll. I don't read magazines or engage others in conversation. I'm focused. I dial the intensity up to a play-off game. The reason I give it my all out there on the exercise floor is because I see it as a matter of life and death.

I have been slaving in the gym for two years, and the structure and appearance of my body are remarkably different from what they were when I arrived home for my first Thanksgiving. With the reintroduction of solid food into my diet, I ratcheted up my fitness program to include anaerobic exercise, which is a form of nonsustained physical activity that typically involves strength training or lifting free weights. Anaerobic exercise puts so much stress on the muscles that all available oxygen is consumed. We are literally forcing the muscles to briefly work in an environment absent of oxygen. I've divided my body into five muscle groups: my chest, my shoulders, my arms, my back, and my legs. I rotate every five days, focusing on one of those body parts with a combination of Nautilus-type machines and the free-weight sets available at the YMCA. In addition, I perform daily stomach crunches and sit-ups.

If you have the money, I would recommend that you hire a personal trainer to guide, encourage, and exhort you into getting into better shape. Even if it's just for a few sessions, a trainer can start you off on the right foot and teach you the appropriate techniques. Personal trainers can motivate you in a million different ways, and the good ones hold you accountable. Personal trainers track your progress, correct your form (since people can injure themselves with improper weight-training techniques), show you new ways to exercise, and stimulate you to give it your all. Making an appointment means you have to show up, unless you're willing to pay a cancellation fee. There's accountability built into this equation.

You know, when you're working out hard on a treadmill or stair-stepper, you see things happening in the gym. What I've observed is people working out like demons for one week and disappearing. It's amazing how many people I have seen come and go at the Palomar Family YMCA.

Don't be a one-week wonder. Remember that you are in this for the long haul and that you won't be able to sustain any weight loss without the exercise component. I've never met nor have I ever treated anyone who lost weight and kept it off without exercising. Not one person.

There are ways you can increase physical activity in your daily routines. Nobody circled more mall parking lots than I did, trying to find that elusive free parking place close to the entrance. I certainly didn't save any time since I could have parked in the back forty and walked to the front entrance in the same amount of time it took me to find a great place. And I could have burned a few calories.

My advice would be for you to *look* for opportunities to park in the back of the lot and hoof it to where you want to go. This means you'll have to wear "sensible shoes," but most women can't wear those stylish high heels to any place but the Junior League ball because they're so uncomfortable to wear.

Another great tip is to wear comfortable sneakers or walking shoes to work and carry a pair of nice shoes in a bag or store a pair in your desk. You can slip on your sneakers to walk to another building, walk fifteen minutes during your morning or afternoon break, or embark on a lunchtime power walk. Climbing stairs is another convenient way to exercise aerobically. The next time a meeting is called, take the stairs instead of the elevator.

Hippocrates, who lived from 460 to 370 BC, is recognized as the father of medicine. You probably knew this was coming, but he was Greek. "All parts of the body which have a function," he said, "if used in moderation and exercised in labors in which each is accustomed, become thereby healthy, well-developed, and age more slowly; but if unused and left idle they become liable to disease, defective in growth, and age quickly."

In his own wise way, Hippocrates was the first to say, "Use it or lose it."

SOME MORE EXERCISE PEARLS

Here are some additional things to keep in mind regarding exercise:

Pearl #1: Make Exercise Pleasurable

If you're not having fun, you will find it very difficult to stay motivated to exercise. Is there something you enjoy doing as you get those legs moving and arms pumping? Is it being outdoors and taking in the beauty of God's nature as you walk? Trying to turn a long single into a double in softball? If you love basketball, join an early morning league. If you like the wind flying in your face, ride a bicycle.

Dancing classes, hiking clubs, and cross-country ski trips are all examples of putting some pleasure into the healthy routine. For some of you, time at the gym might feel like a dungeon of torture. Well, then, find a pool to swim in, a mountain to climb, or a floor to dance on. You gotta shake a leg and cut a rug.

I also bring something more than a towel to the treadmill—I also bring my portable CD player. I have to listen to music that I enjoy. In fact, I get into the music so much that I lose myself, which helps pass the time. Sometimes I pretend the stair-stepper is my dance floor.

You don't have to listen to upbeat music or Greek arias. Audiobooks or talk radio can help the time pass very quickly. Listening to something through my headphones and working hard on an aerobic machine is a great way to redeem lost time. Even the simplest exercise machine comes with a reading rack so that you can read your favorite magazine or finish that book you've been meaning to get to. Just be sure you're working hard enough to drip some sweat on the pages.

High-end fitness clubs even have exercise machines with com-puter screens linked to the Internet so that you can read e-mail or surf the Web. That wouldn't work for me, but if wired technology turns your crank, go for it.

Pearl #2: Shoot for a Goal

After I flew home from Hawaii, I upped the ante by trying to see how low I could go with my weight. To keep myself mentally sharp in the gym, I talked with some good buddies about climbing the highest mountain in the continental United States—Mount Whitney in the California High Sierra. I was told to expect a grueling, oxygen-sapping trek to the top of Whitney, so I prepared by hiking several peaks close to home. The biggest tune-up was tackling San Jacinto Peak outside Palm Springs in the middle of summer with my brother John. We strapped on back-packs and filled them with two-liter bottles of diet soda and water to weigh ourselves down and test our fitness and durability. In the space of six horizontal miles, this stupendous mountain rose from a desert escarpment with an altitude of 1,100 feet to the summit of 10,804-foot San Jacinto Peak. When we reached the top, I knew I was ready.

Trekking up Mount Whitney a month later was easy and practi-cally anticlimactic because of our leisurely, five-day pace. But Mount Whitney served its purpose—it gave me a goal during the summer of 2002 to get into optimal shape, and I was rewarded when I came off that mountain weighing 197 pounds, my low-tide mark.

What would be a good goal for you? It doesn't necessarily have to be running in a 10K race or participating in a half-marathon walk to benefit breast cancer research. You can give yourself a treat (a week-end getaway, a new outfit) for working out thirty consecutive days. Be creative. Shoot for something fun. Maybe it will be a new piece of jewelry or treating yourself to a sports massage.

The art of massage dates back to when the ancient Greeks carried around bottles of scented oil for their daily rubs. A massage increases blood and lymph flow, improves range of motion, helps repair fatigued muscles, and gives your body a glow. So if having someone's trained fingers knead your sore muscles sounds like a wonderful treat, give yourself a realistic goal to shoot for.

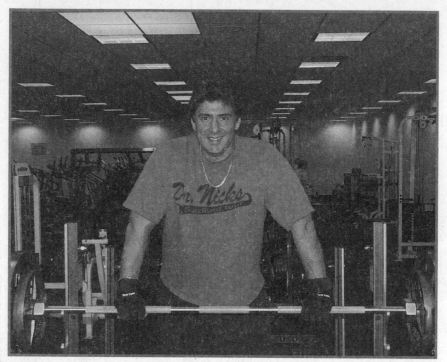

Exercise is a huge component of keeping the weight off these days. I faithfully pump iron at the Palomar Family YMCA in Escondido.

Pearl #3: Share the Pain with a Friend

Having an exercise buddy can make exercise more tolerable and worthwhile. Whether or not you're competitive, it helps to pump a stair-stepper with a friend at your side who can motivate you and even hold you accountable. I have become good friends with a core of the regulars at the Y who have become my exercise comrades.

Make exercise a group experience. Make it a form of family togetherness. Sharing the experience with others helps pass the time, pushes you to work harder, and will motivate you to return for your next workout.

Exercise burns calories. Exercise builds muscle mass, which, in turn, burns even more calories. Burning up the calories in the fuel we consume is what it's all about.

Just do it.

CHAPTER THIRTEEN
PILLAR V:
PLAN A
RADICAL
SABBATICAL

Eighteen months after the Last Supper, my brother John received an interesting phone call. A reporter from the *National Enquirer*—yes, I'm talking about that infamous supermarket tabloid—was looking for me, but my phone number was unlisted. The only Yphantides he could find was my brother John, an estate-planning attorney with his own practice in nearby Rancho Bernardo.

After the reporter relayed his desire to interview me for a story, John immediately called me. "Nick, you'll never believe what just happened."

"Try me," I replied.

"Dude, the *National Enquirer* is interested in doing a story on you. Can you believe that?"

"C'mon, John, get outta here. Are you serious?"

"I just got off the phone with a reporter from the *Enquirer*. Said his name was Philip Smith, and he sounded British. Apparently, somebody from Escondido sent him some newspaper clippings about the trip, and now this guy wants to talk to you."

I shared a good laugh with my brother, but when I hung up the phone, I felt spooked. I could imagine seeing the following headlines at every supermarket checkout in America:

"Elvis Love Child Found Practicing Medicine as a 467-Pound Doc"

or

"Overweight Doc Says Aliens Zapped His Fat on Trip to Mars."

Should I cooperate or not cooperate? My first response was not to return the reporter's inquiry but seek counsel from trusted sources. I called Dad and my pastor, Pat Kenney, and we had lengthy discussions about whether I should cooperate with the *National Enquirer*. At stake was my personal reputation in the community and even around the country. I was concerned about being made an object of mockery. After considering the pros and cons, we reached the conclusion that we should proceed cautiously by investigating what their intentions were.

With some measure of trepidation, I telephoned Philip Smith. "Why would a publication like the *National Enquirer* be interested in a story like mine?" I began.

"My dear sir, are you kidding?" replied Smith in an accent as thick as English marmalade. "This is nothing short of a miracle. This is one of the most amazing things I have ever heard. It's not every day that a 467-pound doctor traipses around the country for eight months and loses 270 pounds going to baseball games. I mean, come on. There's no angle here. We just want to tell your amazing story."

That sounded reasonable to me. "What do you want to know?" I asked, and from there, we proceeded to do a ninety-minute interview. The result was a full-page splash published in the September 10, 2002, edition. With a picture of me standing inside an old pair of size 60 pants and the baseball diamond at Qualcomm Stadium in the background, the snappy headline read: "World Serious: 470-Pound Doc Loses a Whopping 270 Pounds Visiting Every Ball Park in America." What a hoot! I like to shock people by telling them that the *National Enquirer* got the story right, but I have to give credit where credit is due.

The *Enquirer* reporter was especially interested in the baseball angle. "Why did you choose to go around the country watching baseball games?" Smith asked early in our interview. It's a question I'm used to hearing from people vaguely aware of my story.

What I told Smith and anyone who asks is that the genesis of my weight-loss journey began in my patients' examination rooms. Every day, I preached the gospel of good health while practicing it with the profoundest hypocrisy. To get past my patients' natural cynicism—*Yeah, right, Dr. Nick, shape yourself up*—I always had to qualify myself, always had to humble myself, always had to put myself down before I could clear my throat and say something like, "You know, Agnes, the chart says you're one hundred pounds overweight, and if you don't do anything about it . . ."

One day in February 2000, I was particularly discouraged because I was sick and tired of acting like a hypocrite. Then something interesting happened. A friend asked me, "Hey, Nick, are you running for reelection?"

At the time I was serving the last year of a four-year term as chairman of the Palomar Pomerado Health Board, a publicly elected position. I was the Big Daddy, so to speak, also serving as the medical director of a large network of community health clinics with dozens of physicians working under me.

A couple of confidants predicted that I was a rising political star destined to be elected mayor of Escondido or to the California State Assembly—maybe even the U.S. Congress. A *San Diego Union-Tribune* columnist, Logan Jenkins, called me "the most inspiring" candidate in local politics.

What political observers found unique was that my conservative, moral philosophy, combined with a compassionate social agenda, had mass appeal to both sides of the political aisle. Combine that with a disposition of an obese gentle giant, viewed as a larger-than-life advocate for the poor, and you can see why some touted me as someone with a bright political future.

That simple question—"Hey, Nick, are you running for reelection?"—hit me like a torpedo in the midsection of the *Titanic*. For eighteen months, I had been struggling with how to address my morbid obesity following the surgery and radiation therapy for my testicular cancer. The thought of running for reelection to public office and living with my obese condition for an additional four years made me sick. I did the math and projected that when my second term was complete, I would be nearly forty years old and still in the most pitiful and desperate state of physical health. Like lightning through my heart, like an earthquake that brought down my high towers of expectations, my lofty goals for the coming years came tumbling down. I knew it was time to do something about my massive weight.

Over the course of the next eight weeks, I went through much soul-searching and introspection. Believe it or not, I even fasted and prayed. I eagerly sought the counsel of advisers, confidants, family members, and God Himself. I believe the solution came as an answer to prayer when I thought of the novel concept of combining something that I would thoroughly enjoy with something that would be great for my health. *That's it—going around the country drinking protein shakes and watching baseball games.*

Suddenly, the clouds of my heart lifted and my emotions cleared. A determination settled deep within me. In sports lingo, I would put it on the line, let it all hang out, and swing for the fences. I would pursue better health, a lifelong travel dream, and a baseball fantasy during an entire major-league season.

What I did was think of something outside the box to break my loathsome habit of overeating. Habits are hard to break. Lifelong habits are harder to break. Lifelong habits that provide immense pleasure are often impossible to break. My overeating habit had grown to such a magnitude that I had to do something way beyond the ordinary because my health was in such a sorry condition. If I didn't make its restoration the focus of my very existence, I would cease to exist. For one year, I committed to giving up the creature comforts of daily living and putting my medical career on hold, which, up to that time, I had spent more time preparing for than practicing. I knew that was a radical decision, but my life depended on my losing weight and keeping it off for good.

A SABBATICAL FROM THE ORDINARY

That was my thinking when I came up with a plan to travel around the country drinking protein shakes while watching baseball games— something I later called my "Distraction from Deprivation." In true Greek form, I now had my own version of Homer's *Odyssey*. I knew I would eventually get where I wanted to go because I *had* to succeed.

What about you? Have you ever thought about the possibility of taking a sabbatical to restore your most prized possession—your health? The concept of a sabbatical dates back to Genesis, when God created the earth in six days and rested on the seventh. The seventh day of the week became known as the Sabbath. The ancient Jews carried this concept further when they designated every seventh year a sabbatical during which their land remained fallow. Today, when we hear the word *sabbatical,* we think of professors or teachers who take a year to recharge their batteries through travel, writing, and research.

Sabbatical is the right word because those with a significant amount of weight to lose need to step back and take time off from the normal routine. It's getting *out* of the routine that helps you break the cycle of what got you overweight in the first place. As for myself, I understood that a sabbatical would be a welcome rest from a very unhealthy lifestyle of overeating, so I knew I was making the right call. I decided to call this idea a "radical sabbatical."

If you *have* to lose a significant amount of weight, you must seriously consider the notion of a radical sabbatical. I know. The idea sounds preposterous. Your friends will look at you as though you have three eyes, and some may question your mental fitness, but this is something to which you must give some serious thought.

Looking back, I can certainly state that I was so confident I was doing the right thing that when I gave my one-year notice to the Escondido Community Health Center in 2000, it didn't faze me when some of my colleagues wondered if a coconut had fallen on my head. Here's a sampling of their reactions:

- "You've got to be kidding me, Nick. Losing weight while going to baseball games?"
- "Baseball is such a boring sport. Why would anyone go to baseball games except to eat?"
- "Nick, why are you giving everything up and going off on this adventure? Are you joking me?"

I smiled and looked at those people. *I'm glad you're telling me this now because you obviously don't get it.*

My challenge to you is to conduct a personal inventory and decide if a radical sabbatical will work for you. Whether you have twenty pounds or two hundred pounds to lose, taking time off from life may be the breakthrough you need. All other "diets" have failed, right?

I can already hear the objections. *I can't afford a weight-loss sabbatical. It'll cost too much time and too much money.* I'm here to tell you that you can't afford *not* to do it. My health was in such a precarious state that I had a crash-course destiny with premature death. Who cares about owning a house if you're not there to live in it? Who cares about retirement savings if you will not see a single day of retirement? Who cares about your dreams when you won't live long enough to fulfill them?

Pause and contemplate your future. Think and pray about your health dilemma. Carefully consider the magnitude and intensity of the eating-related habits that you must break. I have clearly established that being overweight or being obese is not a matter of snacking on too many Twinkies. It's a complex combination of behavioral, emotional, social, cultural, psychological, and lifestyle issues. Without undergoing a radical sabbatical, you don't give yourself much chance to succeed.

Your radical sabbatical should combine something you love with something you've never had time to do. For guys, it might be traveling to different NFL stadiums during the fall months or following the NASCAR race car circuit during the spring. It could be riding monster roller coasters at different amusement parks during the summer. Maybe it's something as simple as playing golf every day for a month.

For women, a radical sabbatical may be visiting the best shopping meccas in the country, like the Mall of America in Bloomington, Minnesota; Neiman Marcus in Dallas; Cherry Creek in Denver; Rodeo Drive in Los Angeles; or Fifth Avenue in New York City. Perhaps you'd like to be a studio guest for the late-night shows hosted by Jay Leno or Dave Letterman, or travel to Chicago to see Oprah in person.

You could walk across the state, raising money for every pound you lose for a worthy charitable cause. Retrace the John Muir Trail through the High Sierra. The possibilities are endless.

Of course, we have to talk in practicalities. A radical sabbatical depends on your family situation, your job, and your bank account. A mom with two preschoolers at home and one in school can't leave her children or her spouse behind. A father with a good job can't quit or ask for extended time off and still expect his job to be waiting when he returns. Students have to stay in school to earn their degrees.

I would venture that the vast majority of my readers do not have the financial resources to go out on the road for longer than a few days or a week. I admit my situation was very unusual, a "perfect storm" of being single, being able to step away from my medical career, and having enough equity in my home to borrow against it to pay for my weight-loss journey. I spent $50,000 on my radical sabbatical, which doesn't include the lost income from not working.

I was tapped out financially when I arrived home for Thanksgiving, but I was incredibly happy because I knew I would reach my weight-loss goals. I was able to start earning an income as a part-time physician, working enough hours to put salad on the table. I had put *everything* on the line—my health, my career, and my financial future—to lose weight, and that was why I was so determined to see it through. With so much on the line, success was the only option. I had everything to lose—not just the weight.

I want you to experience that same feeling, and you can. If you can't go the radical sabbatical route, shoot for the next best thing. For some of you, that might mean using all your vacation time at once—two to four weeks—to jump-start your weight-loss adventure. Even if you can only get away for one week or a four-day weekend, make it happen. You have to make your radical sabbatical fun. Take a trip. Get out of town. Expand your horizons.

I've come up with three options for your radical sabbatical—Monumental, Moderate, and Minimal. As you read through these, ask yourself which one suits your current lifestyle and present work situation, while taking into consideration how much weight you need to lose:

MONUMENTAL SABBATICAL

Time commitment: Three to twelve months.

Best suited for: Those needing to lose one hundred or more pounds of weight.

Recommended diet: A medically supervised, very low-calorie diet, including liquid protein programs.

Exercise plan: A gym membership starting with walking on a treadmill and consulting with a physical trainer.

Cost: Expensive.

We've already talked about wild and crazy things you can do. Maybe you want to expand your horizons internationally. Have you always wanted to tour the crown capitals of Europe? Be in Cannes during the International Film Festival? Attend tennis's Grand Slam events at Roland Garros in Paris and Wimbledon in London? What about a pilgrimage to a place of spiritual significance, like the Vatican?

If trains, planes, and automobiles turn you off, you can camp yourself—and be pampered—at resorts whose purpose is to help you lose weight. Derided as "fat farms," these all-inclusive resorts provide an oasis-like retreat to help people break the cycle of bad habits. You can find these resorts on the Internet, but if you have to ask how much it costs, you can't afford it.

It is possible to find nice resorts in all price ranges, but even a free stay at your Uncle Bob's lakeshore cabin will work.

MODERATE SABBATICAL

Time commitment: Two weeks to three months.

Best suited for: Those seeking to lose less than one hundred pounds.

Recommended diet: Start with a very low-calorie diet like a liquid protein program, followed by a long-term diet that works for you—Body for Life, South Beach, modified Atkins, Weight Watchers, etc.

Exercise plan: A gym membership plus some form of regular exercise classes.

Cost: Moderate to expensive.

The Moderate Sabbatical could be a miniversion of my baseball tour. Or perhaps you want to develop a new hobby, break 100 on the golf course, or spend concentrated time preparing for a 10K for breast cancer research.

MINIMAL SABBATICAL

Time commitment: A long weekend to two weeks.

Best suited for: Those seeking to lose between twenty and fifty pounds.

Recommended diet: Applying the commonsense suggestions found in Pillar III, in addition to a specific diet that works for you—Body for Life, South Beach, modified Atkins, Weight Watchers, etc.

Exercise plan: Joining a gym or purchasing a used treadmill or stationary bike.

Cost: Modest to moderate.

Even a short-term adventure can help you start new habits, like the elimination of sweets between meals and after dinner, cutting out nondiet sodas, cutting way back on carbs like potatoes, pasta, and rice, and getting used to practicing portion control.

Let me reemphasize how important the exercise component is since physical exertion burns calories. Pillar IV is critical, so if you're a parent with kids, thinking there is just no way you can break away and get some exercise, take heart because you can be creative here as well. My brother John attaches a bicycle trailer to the back of his bike, and now he takes his two young children with him when he goes out on a ride. My sister-in-law, Betsy, has a jogging stroller that she pushes as she either runs or walks with her children. My friend Willy Foster, the ER doc from the Bronx, purchased specially designed backpacks into which he slips his infant adopted daughters from China. He and his wife have gone on overnight backpacking trips with their daughters. For as crazy as it sounds, kids are sturdy. They'll survive. This is about Mommy's or Daddy's survival so the kids won't be left behind as orphans.

A WORD ABOUT LIQUID PROTEIN DIETS

You've probably noticed that I've recommended liquid protein programs for folks in the Monumental and Moderate categories. I think now is a good time to discuss in greater detail what my thinking was when I began my liquid diet.

I haven't mentioned what brand of protein powder I used because I did not want that to be a distraction. In other words, some people think if they just drink supplement shakes, then the pounds will melt away. It's not that simple.

Many diet experts say the ideal pace for permanent weight loss is one pound per week. If you have thirty or fewer pounds to lose, you'll be done in a half year. But when you have more than one hundred pounds to lose as I did, a leisurely weight-loss pace is out of the question. With a weight-loss goal of 270 pounds, I would have been on a diet for more than five years if I took that approach.

I did a lot of research up front in considering all my dietary options. I decided to go for the gusto and to undertake the most aggressive diet I could find. I chose a protein powder that costs an average of $10 a day, which means I spent an easy $2,500 on this diet, but it was worth it. By substituting regular food with protein shakes each day, I cut my caloric intake by 86 percent—from 5,600 to 800 calories per day. One way or another, I was guaranteed success.

This approach is not for everyone, however. There are serious health risks, multiple complications, and significant dollar costs associated with liquid diets such as mine. The program absolutely requires medical supervision and frequent office visits so that your doctor can perform blood tests, check electrocardiograms (EKGs), and closely monitor your vital signs. While medical supervision is necessary for anyone on a liquid diet, it is even more critical for patients being treated for any medical condition. For example, diabetics would require extremely close monitoring, but the drastic weight loss could eventually lead to the resolution of their disease.

Despite the potential downside, I chose the protein shake route for several reasons. Drinking shakes was a detox period, a phase of severe caloric deprivation as I transitioned from one way of living to another. I took a food holiday while I reprogrammed my emotional and mental hard drives. The severe caloric restriction led to significant weight loss right away, which reinforced my good intentions early on. The diet is safe as long as it is appropriately supervised by medical doctors. Another reason I liked it was because it eliminated choice. Oh, I could change the flavor of my shake or what low-calorie drink I mixed it with, but that was the extent of my choice.

This drastic option should be reserved for those with fifty or more pounds to lose. If you believe that a similar liquid diet would be the thing to get you over the hump, then I encourage you to carefully and prayerfully consider starting your radical sabbatical the same way I did. Be sure to work in partnership with your physician when deciding which program is appropriate for you.

For sure, drinking protein shakes is a much better option than gastric bypass surgery, which I will discuss in Chapter 18. Surgery for me was out of the question, so this was the best possible alternative for losing hundreds of pounds and losing them promptly and safely.

Gastric bypass surgery is drastic. I didn't want to get that radical.

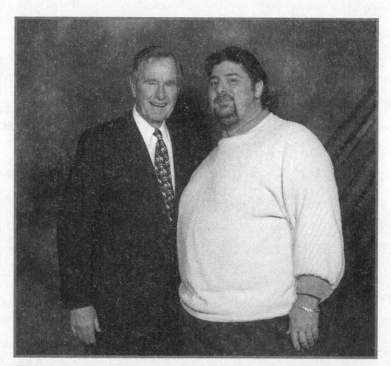

President George Bush is said to have a weakness for pork rinds . . .

CHAPTER FOURTEEN
PILLAR VI: DON'T TRAVEL ALONE

On the Sunday morning before the Last Supper, I was running late for church. I squeezed my bloated body into the Expedition and roared out of the neighborhood until I came to a traffic signal on Valley Parkway.

I missed the green light, so I had to stop. A guy hawking the Sunday paper immediately descended on me. I knew he was part of the Alpha Project, which helps homeless men—who need a hand up, not a handout—by having them hustle newspapers at major intersections. Every copy they sell goes toward their room and board during their comprehensive three-step recovery program.

"Get a newspaper and help the homeless," he pitched. I didn't need a paper since I already subscribed to the *North County Times*. In fact, I had nearly run over my copy in the driveway as I hurried out the door.

I rolled down my window to be friendly.

"Sorry, but I already get the paper at—"

What was a photo of *me* doing on the front page, above the fold?

"Wait a minute," I said. "Can I take a closer look?"

"Sure, mister."

"I'll take five copies," I said, handing him a $10 bill.

"Are you serious?"

"Sure. That's me on the front page," I said, bursting with pride. The feature story was titled "On the Road to Health," and it pictured my bloated self sitting inside the USS *Spirit of Reduction*.

"Holy smokes, that is you," the hawker said. "If I was on the front page of the paper, I'd buy five copies, too."

We'd probably still be joking and bantering if a dozen cars hadn't started honking their horns after the light turned green.

With great excitement, I pulled over to the curb and quickly scanned the article. The reporter, Gig Conaughton, had done a fine job. Then a sobering thought came to mind: *Wait a minute. More than one hundred thousand readers now know that I will be traveling around the country to watch baseball games and lose weight. How can I ever walk the streets of Escondido if I return just as fat as I am today?*

That thought stewed in my mind as I pulled into the church parking lot. As soon as I opened the car door, though, my good friend Mark Searle was pestering me like a Little Leaguer after Sammy Sosa's autograph.

"Can you sign?" he asked, holding out a copy of the front section and a black Sharpie.

"Get out of town, Mark," I replied good-naturedly, knowing he was pulling my big leg. Ever since the local media had found out why I wasn't running for reelection to the local hospital board—to go on this "baseball diet," as they put it—I had been the subject of more than a dozen newspaper and TV feature stories. Several talk-show hosts also invited me to discuss my upcoming trip on their drive-time programs. I never sought the media attention, nor did I have a publicist, but I guess my story was unusual enough that people in the media found it interesting.

Now here's the intriguing aspect to all this. Remember what happened one week later on April Fools' Day when I weighed myself with my brother Phil? To my horror, I learned that I was 467 pounds, not the "roughly 350 pounds" that Gig Conaughton and every reporter had written leading up to the Last Supper.

After Phil confirmed that, yes, I weighed a good hundred pounds more than previously thought, I felt compelled to call Gig and tell him so that the newspaper could run a correction. To me, this was a matter of accountability. I weighed 467 pounds, not 350 or so, and that was the truth. I was willing to be accountable to my family and to my community regarding how much I weighed and how much I lost in the coming months.

In order to succeed, I knew I needed accountability. That's why I asked my brother Phil to oversee my weight-loss journey. That's why I welcomed the press coverage. Now the whole world (well, San Diego County) knew about my upcoming trip, and if I limped back into town still weighing 467 pounds, then I would have been the biggest fool living in the nation's seventh-largest city.

Most people don't like to walk around with dunce caps on their heads, which is why many heavy and obese people aren't interested in being held accountable for losing weight. They are used to eating in secret and dieting in secret. They are used to going through life privately dealing with their obesity. The way they eat in public is not an accurate reflection of their eating behavior behind closed doors.

When they decide to "do something" about the weight, their mind-set is: *I know what I need to do, but I don't want the world knowing that I'm trying to lose weight. What if I fail? Besides, my weight is a very private and personal matter.* As such, they start and stop their weight-loss efforts locked in a closet of veiled anonymity. By flying solo, it deprives them of the opportunity to be victorious and robs family and friends of responding and participating. It's as if they are preparing themselves for defeat. As Winston Churchill once said, "Victory finds a hundred fathers, but defeat is an orphan."

Though I will acknowledge that my story has unique circumstances, the principle of accountability and reliance on others is universally applicable to your situation. The realization that you—and only you—are responsible for what happens when you attempt to lose weight does make you vulnerable. I strongly feel, however, that deliberately placing yourself in a position of being accountable to others is an absolute necessity.

For you to succeed with accountability, you will need to:

Have a Travel Companion

When you start your weight-loss journey, I implore you not to travel alone. Have family and friends around as much as possible; you're less likely to wander off the reservation when someone close to you is aware of what you should and shouldn't be doing to accomplish your goals. You need someone to be your cheerleader and someone with whom you can share your temptations and even your failures.

For most of my trip, with very little exception, I had someone sitting shotgun in the USS *Spirit of Reduction*. At various times, my father George, my grandfather John Pfaff, my pastor Pat Kenney, and my good friends Dr. Donald Miller, Jose "Chuy" Escobedo, and Mike Grant were among the dozen or so who joined me on the road. I knew I couldn't cheat when I was in their presence.

These individuals loved and cared for me enough to come alongside me as human pillars of support and encouragement. During the darkest days of my initial transition—that first week—my father was the right man at the right time. He put up with the short-tempered outbursts, the nasty frustrations, and the negative and critical spirit that passed through my body during the early detoxification process. Dad was a constant source of support, motivation, and affirmation. He did so with a selfless attitude of love and compassion.

While it's doubtful that you'll be taking an RV trip as I did, you're still going on a journey, so it's imperative to find individuals you love and respect to come alongside you. Give access to the inner sanctum of your heart. Allow others the opportunity to participate and encourage you as you travel on your weight-loss adventure.

I recommend that accountability go beyond one person. The weight of your situation means that it takes more than a single individual to carry the load. Your accountability partners should feel comfortable asking you the tough questions:

- "Are you sticking to your diet?"
- "What have you eaten today?"
- "Have you been snacking on things you shouldn't have?"
- "How much did you weigh at your last weigh-in?"
- "Are you still resolved to see this thing through?"

You want your accountability partners to know that you're on a diet, what your weight is, how much weight you've lost, how much weight you've gained, and whether you're staying on track. You should also give them the right to transmit that information to others.

Some of you may not have even one person you feel comfortable to ask to help you out. Perhaps you've just moved to a new community, or you have strained family relationships, or maybe your marriage is on the rocks.

If this sounds like you, the answer is a support group. Nearly all communities and larger churches have them; it's just a matter of making the necessary inquiries to find them. An established group like Overeaters Anonymous is a great place to start, or your local hospital may have support groups in conjunction with medically supervised weight-loss programs.

Whatever form it takes, you need to find accountability. I recommend that it starts from the very first weigh-in. When I started my diet on April Fools' Day, I had nothing to hide from Phil. I had taken off my clothes and stood naked before my brother. That type of accountability could have been humiliating and embarrassing, but I saw it as liberating. I was finally free from the lies and misrepresentation of how much I ate, and that was a very empowering experience that changed my life. I know accountability can change your life, too.

Make Your Accountability Sacrificial

I am amazed when I hear people say, "I could never afford to do what you did." Sure, some would say that I took a huge financial risk, but I didn't see it that way. My weight-loss odyssey wasn't an irresponsible decision but a calculated financial sacrifice to get back my health. The same people who express wonder at my audacity are often one heartbeat away from dropping dead from a heart attack. I wonder how they could afford not to do it.

Whenever I'm in Las Vegas for a medical conference, I walk through the casinos where I see blackjack tables with a minimum bet of $1,000. I have also seen tables where the minimum bet is $2. You may not need to put up a $0 bet like I did on the blackjack table of life, but you need to put up something. How much are you willing to risk to become healthy? How many chips are you willing to push into the center of the table?

Lifestyle reengineering, lifestyle redesign, creating new habits, unwiring or deprogramming old habits, being accountable to others, spending daily time working out—all these require time. Time is by far my most precious commodity, as I'm sure it is for you as well. If you think you don't have extra time, let me ask you this:

- Have you ever considered working thirty hours a week?
- Have you ever considered downsizing your house and your body simultaneously?
- Have you ever thought about getting a new job as you start a new life?

Only you in your heart can know what kind of commitment it will take to change the way you see so that you can change the way you look. Making yourself accountable by making some bold sacrifices as part of your weight-loss journey will go a long way in helping you stay on course.

Be Willing to Go Public Beyond Your Family and Friends

In preparation for my weight-loss journey, I started a Web site with the idea of using it to keep family and friends updated on my journey and my progress. I posted pictures from my digital camera and composed lengthy update letters every couple of weeks. Having my own Web site sure beat licking stamps for postcards.

An unexpected thing happened. My little Web site (health steward.com) started exploding with hits from total strangers as word of mouth spread about this four-hundred-plus-pound doc crisscrossing America with a protein shake in his right hand. I can't express how humbled I felt when I logged on to my computer each day and found dozens of e-mails waiting for me from people I had never met. Their e-mails and feedback became a source of inspiration to me.

Suddenly, my desire to keep family and friends informed of my progress had become something much greater. There were obese people out there in cyberspace depending on me for advice and encouragement. The sense of accountability deepened even further. Now there was more at stake than just my waistline, and it all started with my willingness to be accountable and transparent with my journey.

People respond to transparency, so I recommend that you send updates via an e-mail "blast" to family and friends when you begin your own radical sabbatical. If you can set up a Web site (or have a friend do that for you), that's even better. Other ideas include writing your own weight-loss newsletter, creating your own weight-loss support group, joining an online weight-loss community, committing yourself to an Internet-based chat forum, or starting a church-based weight-loss group.

Be an Accountability Partner to Others

These principles apply in both directions. Being the source of support to others you know on their own weight-loss journey will raise your spirits. Be sure to match emotion for emotion. I knew that when obese people poured out their hearts and frustrations to me, they deserved a matching response. I wrote back long e-mails, telephoned some, and gave warm hugs whenever we met in person.

I'm proud that I answered every single e-mail during my eight months on the road. I fear that I will not be able to keep up when *My Big Fat Greek Diet* is released, but it won't be for a lack of effort. I'm willing to help out because I knew that I could not do this on my own, and neither can you.

Consider the Role of Divine Accountability

As if it's not obvious already, I have a confession to make. The cornerstone of my motivation is the accountability I have to a personal and loving God.

The initial spark that ignited the forest fire of determination in my heart came because of a very simple revelation. When I had to face my physical mortality as a human being, I discovered something very profound. Cancer made me realize that my physical health is a God-given gift. As such, it is my conviction and belief that I have the responsibility to honor God in return by being a good caretaker of that gift. I call this personal health stewardship.

It is my desire to be a good steward—a good caretaker—of this miraculous gift called life. I'm convinced that living life in the manner that life's very Designer intended it to be lived is the best thing I could do with my existence. God's way is the best way. God's design is a miraculous design. God's plan is an amazing plan.

I know now that God's perfect plan for me was never to weigh 467 pounds. My failure to honor God in caring for His temple within me was something that convicted me. Once I determined to start on April 1, I became very committed to changing. With the greatest sense of appreciation, I declare my intention to care for His personal gift of life to me.

It is my prayer that you, too, will come to truly grasp what a priceless gift your personal health really is. By getting in shape you'll honor God, and the benefits of doing so will go way beyond the physical realm. Trust me, I know.

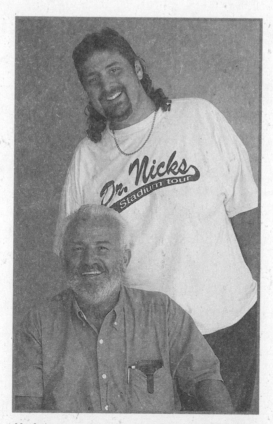

My father was there for me—especially during my first week, when I nearly quit my Big Fat Greek Diet.

CHAPTER FIFTEEN

PILLAR VII: REALIZE THAT YOUR WEIGHT-LOSS JOURNEY IS FOR A LIFETIME

W hy do so many people regain the weight they lose?

That's the question of the ages in the weight-loss world.

I couldn't have told you why before I started my weight-loss odyssey. The most optimistic studies I've seen show that 80 percent of those who lose weight do not manage to keep off the pounds; other studies put that figure at a more pessimistic 95 percent. I generally believe that 90 percent of all diets fail.

After I caught that 103-pound halibut in Alaskan waters and *knew* victory was in my grasp, I finally understood that temporary deprivation was not the answer to a lifelong dilemma. What was happening to me was a total lifestyle change in the way I ate, what I ate, and how much I exercised.

That's why I've said all along that diets don't work. A diet, by definition, is a regulated selection of food in order to lose weight. If all you're doing is temporarily regulating your intake—with your focus being on the day your diet ends so that you can go to your favorite buffet restaurant and celebrate—what's the point?

People regain their weight because they return to their old habits. Oftentimes because of having undergone a period of deprivation, they overcompensate and eat even more enthusiastically when they are "off" the diet. They end up gaining even more weight than they had lost in the first place.

George Dill, a retired engineer in San Diego, has graciously allowed me to illustrate this point by telling his story. I met George through my father, and he's a little younger than Dad. George happened to own a deli, and as my father would tell you, you can never have too many friends in the deli business.

A couple of years before my baseball tour, Dad said I had to meet George Dill. Apparently, Dad's friend had lost well over one hundred pounds on a liquid fast program supervised by his local HMO. The engineer slimmed down from 340 pounds to a relatively svelte 222 pounds in less than a year, and he hoped to lose forty more pounds to be at his ideal weight.

My father invited him to our house one Sunday afternoon for some *koinonia* and to force-feed some inspiration to a captive audience—me.

"You listen to George," my father instructed moments before his friend's arrival. "This man can teach you something. Look at what he's accomplished."

I was already tired of the harangue. "Dad, I know what I need to do," I said. "I just need to do it. So lay off, would you? Get off my back."

Despite being frustrated, I was appreciative of George's willingness to give up a Sunday afternoon to help me out. After the introductions, we sat out on our back patio while Mom offered him baklava, a Greek delicacy. I was too embarrassed to eat in front of him, so I just listened.

George had brought a thick notebook filled with "before" pictures, charts and graphs documenting his weight loss, and all sorts of weight-loss curriculum. He had received the notebook, which was more like a patient manual, from his doctor.

I remember being very impressed with this outspoken, articulate, and friendly acquaintance of my father's. He gave me a ray of hope that if he could do it, then by George, I could do it as well.

Two and a half years later, I triumphantly returned home for Thanksgiving and my first meal of solid food in eight months. George had seen me featured on KUSI TV, so he was naturally curious to see me again and ask how the trip went.

He called a couple of weeks after Thanksgiving and suggested that we hike Escondido's tallest peak, Bernardo Mountain. It's a half-day trip up and down, and you get a good workout. I thought it was a splendid idea.

Here's the exchange when we met in the parking lot next to the trailhead:

Nick: "George, what happened?"

George: "Nick, what happened to you?"

Nick: "I did what I was supposed to do. What did you do?"

George: "I did what I was *not* supposed to do."

While I had lost weight, George had gained seventy pounds back. Now he was threatening to pass the three-hundred-pound barrier. Despite his weight gain, he was still in good shape, and I huffed and puffed to keep up with him. During our long hike, he told me that he loved to eat more than anything else. He said that when he and his wife took a once-in-a-lifetime trip to Australia and New Zealand, he "fell off the wagon" by enjoying sumptuous meals in nice restaurants. He thought he could chow down 5,000 calories a day but make up for his epicurean indulgence by running three miles a day. Alas, George's metabolism had changed in his midfifties, and running three miles a day wasn't enough to keep the pounds from returning to his midsection.

Regaining the weight wasn't a big deal to him, however. He even played with my mind. "Don't worry," he said. "By next year, you'll be right back where you were. Just you wait. You'll find out how hard it is to keep those pounds off."

That kind of talk depressed me. Hanging out with George made me feel like he would jinx me. It reminded me of a line in *Godfather III*, where Michael Corleone (Al Pacino) exclaims through clenched teeth, "Just when I thought I was out, they pull me back in."

When you start losing weight—making a real impact on the way you look—there will be people telling you in your face that you're going to fail. I'm not telling you to get new friends, but when you were heavy, you probably hung out with friends who liked to eat, who were heavier than average, and who now will look for ways to get in their little digs. They'll say things like, "You may think you're hot stuff now, but you just wait. You'll see."

On the other hand, you may be encouraged by well-meaning friends who feel compelled to warn you about the dangers of going back to your old habits. They may challenge you to stay with the program. George and I have remained friends, and I'm helping poor old George get with a program he can stick with. He thought, as many dieters do, that once he got his weight down, he could return to *la dolce vita*—eating megameals each day. Obviously, that could not happen. He needs to change the way he sees before he can change the way he looks.

SHOW DETERMINATION

No matter whether your friends are cutting or are in your corner, you're going to have to show them.

Show them that you know your weight-loss journey will last a lifetime.

Show them that you have what it takes—mentally, physically, and spiritually—to go the distance.

I knew going in that losing weight was not the battle. Keeping it lost is what it's all about. In my entire life, I have met only one person who has lost more than one hundred pounds and kept it off, and that is my inspirational friend Brad Wiscons, whom I invited over to my home after the first week of my baseball tour. Unfortunately, 99 percent of the people I know who lost much weight gained it all back—and more.

Even before I lost 270 pounds, my focus had always been on what

I would do once I lost the weight. I truly was consumed with this thought because I had seen so many others fall by the wayside and gain it all right back.

I will confess that I was giddy with excitement when I went from looking like an unemployed NFL lineman to a member of a boy band, but deep in my heart, I knew the real show began when I ate solid food on Thanksgiving Day. I knew the Monday mornings when I triumphantly stepped onto a single scale—pretending it was the medals podium at the Olympic Games—would soon be over. The weeks of losing four, five, and seven pounds were history. The days of positive reinforcement as I saw the graph line for my weight steadily go down would soon end. What lay ahead was a graph line that remained horizontal, if I practiced the concepts found in the Seven Pillars.

That line ticked up slightly following my conquest of Mount Whitney, when I weighed 197 pounds. When I look at the photos from that momentous day, I can honestly say that I looked skinny. Believe me, I never thought I'd hear anyone put the adjective *skinny* in front of my name.

I've since gained thirteen pounds or so, but, more important, that graph line has remained as straight as the Pacific horizon off San Diego. With the grace of God, I hope and pray that line doesn't ever budge.

If I need inspiration to see this thing through for a lifetime, I'll remember the story of my father immigrating to America. He came by boat from Athens to New York in 1955 because he couldn't afford the expensive airfare.

For eleven days, Dad endured seasickness in a closet-sized room he shared with another man. By the time he stepped onto American soil, he was happy to leave the sickness behind him and begin a new life. He desperately wanted to succeed in a country where the possibilities were endless.

That's the same attitude you must have. After all the deprivation, all the hard exercise, and all the determination to lose those pounds, you don't want to go back to where you came from. You want to stay where you are and begin a new life.

Would you be reading this book if I gained my weight back? Would you come hear me speak if my story was about a doctor who lost 270 pounds and gained 300 back?

Of course not. I'm motivated to stay at 210 pounds because I don't want to blow my integrity. That motivation comes from Jesus' words found in Matthew 5:16 (CEV): "Make your light shine, so that others will see the good that you do."

My advice for you is to let your light shine before others as they see that your weight-loss journey is for a lifetime.

Finally, the message of Pillar VII is this: Don't start losing weight until you're ready to start a new life. Don't start your journey unless you're willing to live it until you meet your Maker. Don't even think about losing weight until you're ready to leave your current life behind. As challenging and intimidating as the prospect of weight loss may appear, losing the weight is not the issue. Making the changes to make weight loss a permanent part of your reality is what this is all about.

When I came home that Thanksgiving, I knew what I had to do: give away all my old clothes because I was never going *there* again. I had more than a dozen black garbage bags filled with pants in sizes 50, 52, 54, 56, 58, and 60. I had shirts big enough to use as spinnakers on San Diego Bay. There were enough clothes in those garbage bags to stock the large men's department of a local thrift shop.

I had kept those clothes for years because I always expected to lose weight eventually. Now I had blown right past those sizes, and I could fit into pants with a 36-inch waist. So I organized all those unneeded clothes—some barely worn since they didn't fit me for very long— and donated them to a prison ministry called Brother's Keepers, which helps men transition out of prison.

I donated my entire wardrobe except for the following items:

- a dapper navy blue blazer, size 64
- a pair of white slacks, size 60
- a white dress shirt, size XXXXXL

I have determined in my mind that I will never wear those clothes again—until I'm invited to appear on *Oprah*.

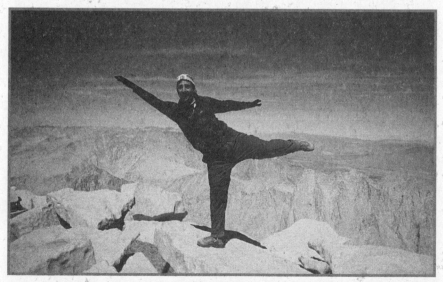

Eighteen months after I began my weight-loss journey, I celebrated my life atop the highest peak in the continental U.S.—Mt. Whitney in California's High Sierra.

PART III

MY BIG FAT GREEK DIET

SIDE DISHES

CHAPTER SIXTEEN

THE FIRST AND LAST WORD IN FAST FOOD

N ow that you have the Seven Pillars under your belt, let's move into some specific areas of tantamount importance— fast food, childhood obesity, and gastric bypass surgery. We'll deal with these topics in that order.

If you live east of the San Andreas Fault, chances are that you've never heard of In-N-Out Burger, a family-owned fast-food chain concentrated in Southern California that has gained a cultlike following for its simple yet classic menu. Ever since In-N-Out opened its first hamburger stand in a Los Angeles suburb back in 1948—seven years before McDonald's was a gleam in Ray Kroc's eye—they have offered only four items: hamburgers, fries, milk shakes, and soft drinks. No namby-pamby grilled chicken sandwiches served at In-N-Out. Instead, juicy and great-tasting burgers are cooked fresh to order. French fries are sliced up from fresh whole potatoes, and shakes are made from real ice cream. You get the picture.

One of the charms of In-N-Out is that you can order items "off menu." Back when I was as rotund as a sumo wrestler, I used to stop at an In-N-Out after a long day of seeing patients and order a "4-by-4"—four hamburger patties and four slices of cheese stacked on top of each other in a single bun. I also asked for large fries and a diet soda—as if choosing a diet drink somehow justified the mouthwatering indulgence.

In my mind, the 4-by-4 was a fast-food work of art, and I regarded this taste treat much as an art lover regards the Mona Lisa: Both were worthy of veneration. If you had told me that a single 4-by-4 contained 1,600 calories and a whopping 108 grams of fat, that nutritional information wouldn't have fazed me at all. A high-calorie, high-fat cheeseburger meant high taste to me.

That's why I often found myself sitting in an In-N-Out drive-thru line after work, my taste buds salivating as my SUV inched toward the pickup window. The way I saw it, a 4-by-4 and fries at 6 p.m. was a great snack to hold me over—until *dinnertime*.

That's really how I viewed meals on the go. In my mind, I never really ate fast food—I *snacked* on it. I led such a busy lifestyle that fast food was something to hold me over between patient visits and running to meetings and community functions.

I ate fast food so often—probably five or six times a week—that my Ford Expedition was literally a fast-food restaurant on wheels. Whenever I happened to be driving to the clinic or the hospital or the university, my SUV gravitated toward fast-food drive-thru lanes like a go-kart following the track at Disneyland's Autotopia. I frequented so many fast-food restaurants that I became a Connoisseur of Grease, a Duke of Burger, if you will. I knew what I liked.

My love for fast food grew as my waistline expanded in my twenties and early thirties. If I happened to drive through a Burger King, for instance, I always ordered the Double Whopper with Cheese Combo, which came with supersized fries and a soft drink. At Wendy's, I was partial to the Triple Decker. At Mickey D's, a Big Mac and a Double Quarter Pounder got the call.

I loved ethnic fast food as well, especially Mexican. In San Diego, most people flock to one of the "Three R's": Rico's, Rubio's, or Roberto's. I preferred Alberto's, however, a hole-in-the-wall where I usually ordered two gut bombs—a carnitas burrito *and* a carne asada burrito, both with extra *queso*. (That's a pork burrito and a steak burrito with extra cheese, for you Midwesterners.) If I wasn't in Alberto's neighborhood, Taco Bell could do in a pinch. I liked ordering a "sleeve" of burritos—a 7-Layer, a Supreme Chicken, and a Supreme Steak.

I could also find Greek fast food at Tom's Burgers, a Southern California chain owned by a Greek family. (Dad knew the family, of course.) I imagine that you're wondering how a place named "Tom's Burgers" could serve Greek food, but Tom's produced great-tasting gyro and pastrami sandwiches, along with the all-American burger topped with chili and extra cheese.

When the chips were down—like when I was diagnosed with testicular cancer—I liked eating KFC's extra-crispy chicken. The extra batter on each breast, leg, thigh, and wing was finger-lickin' good. Other times I would drop by buffets like Hometown Buffet or Souplantation, where I would put one leaf of lettuce on my plate and pile a half pound of potato salad, a half pound of macaroni salad, and a teaspoon of cottage cheese on top. Then I would dump a pile of nuts, bacon bits, and croutons over the mound of food and drown it with several ladles of creamy blue cheese or ranch dressing. My "salad" probably had more calories than three or four hamburgers, but, like many Americans, I wasn't paying attention to calories or fat grams. I just wanted a lot of great-tasting food at a reasonable price.

MEALS ON WHEELS

Great-tasting food at a reasonable price. That pretty much sums up the mission statement of the United States fast-food industry, although some would claim that "great-tasting fast food" is an oxymoron. Still, people vote with their stomachs as well as their feet, and the last time I checked, people were still knocking down the doors of the tens of thousands of fast-food restaurants in this country, so the food can't be *that* bad. As I heard one expert put it: "Americans talk healthy but eat tasty."

No doubt about it: Fast food is *huge* in this country. How huge? Putting your arms around this conglomeration would be like trying to get your arms around my midsection during the Last Supper: I don't think it can be done because it's too massive.

Seventy million Americans each *day*—one-fourth the U.S. population—frequent a fast-food restaurant, a staggering number that is 33 percent *more* than twenty-five years ago. Americans spent more than $110 billion on fast food in 2002, an astronomical amount that's more than what we expended on books, magazines, newspapers, videos, and recorded music combined. McDonald's is the nation's largest purchaser of beef, pork, and potatoes and the second-largest purchaser of chicken, according to author Eric Schlosser, author of *Fast Food Nation: The Dark Side of the All-American Meal.*

Whether we're talking about a behemoth like McDonald's or an upstart like Chipotle, fast-food restaurants are as common as streetlights and found on every main boulevard and commercial thoroughfare in America. Heavily marketed through ad campaigns, movie tie-ins, and celebrity endorsements, fast food saturates TV advertising with jingles that push our hot buttons:

- "You deserve a break today."
- "Have it your way."
- "Buy a bucket of chicken and have a barrel of fun."
- "Make a run for the border."

Do you hear what I'm saying? We're hooked on fast food, prisoners of appetites conditioned to savor all sorts of food items fried in hot oil. Most fast food has more calories per bite than plain home cooking, which is where the hook is set. And it's cheap. With the price-cutting "Burger Wars"—Big Macs and Whoppers for a buck—fast food is regarded as a good deal.

Fast food is readily available everywhere you drive. Stores open before dawn and don't close until late at night, if they shutter their drive-thru windows at all. Millions of commuters start their day with Egg McMuffins, Krispy Kremes, Dunkin' Donuts, or Einstein Bagels. At noontime, white-collar workers empty business parks and flood nearby streets in search of burgers and burritos on the cheap. At the end of the day, working moms pick up hungry kids after soccer practice and Cub Scouts and piano lessons and make a beeline for the drive-thru lane.

Morning, noon, and night, we march into fast-food restaurants like mind-numbed robots, blissfully ordering artery-clogging and indigestion-producing "value meals," unaware—or unwilling—to consider how unhealthy and fattening this food can be. I'm not pointing any fingers because I was Exhibit 1A. Back in my bad old days, I knew that fast food was high in calories and fat grams, but I ate it anyway because it tasted good.

I think everyone knows that fast food is not as healthy as "regular" food, but in recent years we've seen plaintiffs come forward who claim—with a straight face—that they didn't know fast food wasn't good for them. I hate to be the bearer of bad news, but a lifetime of cheeseburgers, crispy chicken sandwiches, thick-crust pizza, carnitas burritos, garlic fries, and thick chocolate shakes will make you as fat as the Goodyear blimp.

That would be news to Caesar Barber, a fifty-seven-year-old blue-collar worker from the Bronx. Barber sued McDonald's, Burger King, Wendy's, and KFC in 2002 for jeopardizing his health with greasy, salty fare. His class-action lawsuit in New York State on behalf of other obese and ill New Yorkers said that the fast-food industry had an obligation to warn consumers of the dangers of eating from their menus.

In his complaint, Barber said he was unaware that eating McDonald's hamburgers four or five times a week wasn't the healthiest thing for his body. He described how his weight ballooned up to 270 pounds (he stood five feet ten inches tall) on a steady diet of Big Macs before he suffered a heart attack. He was trying to sue the pants off Ronald McDonald and other fast-food companies for allegedly contributing to his obesity and subsequent ill health.

Thankfully, this frivolous suit was thrown out of court in 2003, but that won't be the last time we'll see someone trying to convince a judge that the fast-food industry has knowingly contributed to the problem of obesity in America. I predict that we will see more attorneys and consumer activists blaming fast food for the nation's obesity problems. I also predict that we will see the fast-food giants making an effort to serve healthier fare to stave off those lawsuits. I'm sure that's why McDonald's decided to eliminate supersize portions for their fries and drinks by the end of 2004.

GETTING A GRIP ON FAST FOOD

Since fast food is so popular, any discussion on how to lose weight must address our eat-on-the-go culture. I don't think you have to give up fast food completely as you try to lose weight, but you certainly have to think intentionally each time you pull up to the drive-thru lane or step up to the counter to order something to eat.

If you're going to be eating at a fast-food restaurant, you have to walk in with a strategy. Here are a few ideas:

- **Pay close attention to the lower-fat, lower-carbohydrate, lower-calorie items on the menu—and order those.** You may be thinking, *Well what's left?* You can find a few things to eat. I would recommend that you go to my Web site at healthsteward.com, where I provide links to Internet sites that reveal the nutritional breakdown of your favorite fast-food items. (You can also request this information on your next visit to the fast-food restaurant in question, or you can purchase an inexpensive booklet with information at drugstores or bookstores.) Then look for the lower-fat, lower-calorie items.

Because of my modified Atkins' approach, I shy away from white-bread buns and the white-flour "wraps" that seem to be popular today. Almost without fail, I order my hamburgers without a bun, and some fast-food restaurants are quite creative in this area. At In-N-Out, for instance, you can ask for a "protein burger," which is a hamburger wrapped in iceberg lettuce. It's tasty and has 38 percent fewer calories than a regular hamburger. Hardee's and Carl's Jr. now offer "low-carb" burgers and chicken sandwiches wrapped in lettuce, and I predict that many more fast-food chains will follow their lead. I'm still waiting for one of the major pizza chains to come out with a whole-wheat, low-carb crust option, but I feel that's just a matter of time.

- **Make sure that if it fries, it dies.** Breaded or deep-fried fish and chicken sandwiches, topped with a sauce, will have more calories and fat than a plain hamburger. If you happen to eat something like KFC fried chicken (Original Recipe or Extra Crispy), you can peel away the skin and just eat the meat to save yourself a boatload of calories, fat, and carbohydrates. But it's not easy peeling away the great-tasting skin, so you'd be better off buying a piping hot broiled chicken at the supermarket and not tempting yourself.

- **Stay away from the bacon.** As a way to introduce something new and exciting to their menu, fast-food chains have been tossing strips of bacon willy-nilly on their hamburgers and chicken sandwiches. Repeat after me: Bacon is a no-no! Here's an example: A Jack in the Box Double Cheeseburger has 410 calories and 22 grams of fat. A Bacon Bacon Cheeseburger has 910 calories and 59 grams of fat. And the Bacon Ultimate Cheeseburger has 1,120 calories and 75 grams of fat.

- **Don't say "cheese."** Adding cheese to a burger generally adds 40 percent more fat. The more lettuce and tomato that end up between your bun and burger, the more healthy your sandwich will be.

- **Hold the sauce.** Many fast-food chains slap some "secret" sauce on their burgers. That secret sauce is usually a mixture of Thousand Island dressing and ketchup. Stick to regular condiments (ketchup and mustard) if you must. Creamy sauces on chicken sandwiches and tartar sauce with fish are other things to avoid.

- **Say no to "supersize."** The teen behind the counter has been coached to say two things when you step up to order: "Is this for here or to go?" and "Would you like to supersize your meal?" Sure, you get more bang for your buck with the supersized version, but you also receive a corresponding higher number of calories and fat. What you could do if you're trying to eat less *and* be frugal is to order a supersized value meal and split it with a friend. (I'm not talking about sharing a diet cola. Buy an extra one or drink a free water.)

- Remember that anything served with chicken will probably have less fat and less calories than beef. Unless you're ordering a "crispy" chicken sandwich, baked or broiled chicken will contain fewer fat grams than hamburgers. A chicken burrito for example, has roughly half the fat of a carne asada or carnitas burrito.

- Go for the pita sandwiches. More and more fast-food chains have some sort of pita item on their menu these days, and they have significantly fewer calories and fat than regular fare.

- Don't forget that sandwich shops are probably going to be your best bet. Places such as Quizno's, Subway, and Schlotzsky's Deli offer tasty chicken and turkey sandwiches that average 6 grams of fat. Some people have even lost more than a hundred pounds eating fast-food sandwiches (I tell Jared Fogle's story later in this chapter.) If whole grain or whole wheat bread options are available, by all means, order those.

- Order a salad. It's hard to go wrong with a salad, but your dressing should be no-cal or low-cal. If a low-cal dressing is not available, use enough dressing to flavor the salad. Be careful, though. A Taco Salad with salsa from Taco Bell has 380 calories and 42 fat grams because the veggies and cheese arrive in a fried flour taco shell; the shell-less version (or not eating the shell) has exactly half the calories and half the fat.

- **Don't eat everything you bring to the table.** Order a minimal amount of food, eat until you're full, and then doggie-bag or toss the leftovers.

- **Order with your mind, not your stomach.** You have to keep your head when you step up to the counter. Order only what makes sense vis-à-vis the number of calories, fat, and carbohydrates that you're limiting yourself to each day.

All of these principles could easily be applied to any of your favorite local restaurants. Here are some examples of what I would order in some of the popular fast-food chains:

DR. NICK'S PICKS

Jack in the Box

Chicken Teriyaki Bowl: 550 calories and 3 grams of fat
Side Salad: 50 calories and 3 grams of fat (with Low-Calorie Italian Dressing)

McDonald's

Chicken McGrill (without mayo): 300 calories and 6 grams of fat
McSalad Shaker Grilled Chicken Caesar Salad with Fat-Free Herb Vinaigrette: 135 calories and 2.5 grams of fat

Subway

Seven Under 6 Ham Sandwich: 290 calories and 5 grams of fat
Seven Under 6 Veggie Delite: 230 calories and 3 grams of fat

KFC

Honey BBQ Sandwich: 298 calories and 6 grams of fat

Tender Roast Sandwich Without Sauce: 270 calories and 6 grams of fat

Taco Bell

Fiesta Burrito Chicken: 370 calories and 12 grams of fat

Soft Taco Chicken: 190 calories and 6 grams of fat

Carl's Jr. or Hardee's

Charbroiled BBQ Chicken Sandwich: 290 calories and 3.5 grams of fat

Charbroiled Chicken Salad-to-go with Fat-Free Italian Dressing: 215 calories and 7 grams of fat

Burger King

Chicken Whopper (without mayo): 420 calories and 9 grams of fat

BK Veggie Burger (without mayo): 290 calories and 7 grams of fat

THE FAST-FOOD DIET

You want to know the power of TV?

I found out when people started confusing me with Jared Fogle, the guy on the Subway commercials. "So, you lost a lot of weight just like the Subway guy," some people said to me. "Is that because you ate all those Subway sandwiches?" No, I didn't do the "Subway diet," as the media has called it.

Here's what happened. A few years ago, Jared Fogle was a twenty-one-year-old, six-foot, two-inch Indiana University student who weighed 435 pounds. Like me, Jared had a sixty-inch waist and a burning desire to do something about his obesity. The trouble was that he wasn't sure how to go about it. Every diet had failed him.

One day, while Jared was walking to school from his apartment, he passed a Subway restaurant along the way. A sign in the window advertised Subway's new line of sandwiches with less than 6 grams of fat.

Jared came up with a novel plan: lose weight by eating Subway sandwiches. You may be scratching your head and wondering how that worked, but Jared figured that eating two Subway sandwiches a day—for a total of 1,000 calories a day—would start him down the road toward weight loss.

Beginning in March 1998, Jared's daily menu consisted of:

- Breakfast: a cup of coffee
- Lunch: a six-inch turkey sub without mayo and cheese, a bag of Baked Lays chips, and a diet soft drink
- Dinner: a twelve-inch veggie sub without mayo and cheese and a diet soft drink

Jared loaded his sandwiches with tons of lettuce, green peppers, banana peppers, jalapeño peppers, pickles, and a bit of spicy mustard. The question I have is how Jared withstood the monotony of eating the same two Subway sandwiches a day for one year, but maybe that goes to show you how determined he was. Then again, I drank protein shakes every day for eight months, so I guess you gotta do what you gotta do.

Jared also introduced a regimen of walking exercise into his diet (1.5 miles a day) and eventually dropped 245 pounds. His sixty-inch waist shrank to thirty-four inches. His friends and fellow students at Indiana University were amazed by the transformation, which elicited a feature article on him in the student newspaper. The Associated Press and *Men's Health* magazine picked up the story, and when someone at the Subway Corporation read it, the rest became history. Subway decided that Jared would be a great spokesman for its "Low Fat Choices—Seven Under 6 Grams of Fat" sandwich line, so they hired him for a series of advertising campaigns. He became a minor celebrity and appeared on TV talk shows, and I'm pleased that his story has motivated others to lose weight. Best of all, a slimmed-down Jared married his sweetheart, Elizabeth Christie, and he reportedly maintains his weight loss by eating a normal diet of about 2,400 calories a day.

The "Jared diet" isn't for everybody, but it points to a fundamental concept that's applicable to anyone seeking to lose weight: You have to drastically lower the number of calories that your body consumes. And when you're in a fast-food restaurant—for whatever reason— you must stick with the lower-in-calorie, lower-in-fat items and practice portion control. You have to order the right food, eat it for the right reason, and eat the right amount.

I'll never forget the first time my cowriter, Mike Yorkey, and I met to discuss this book. We happened to huddle up over lunchtime at an In-N-Out Burger restaurant close to my home.

Isn't that why anyone goes to a fast-food restaurant—for the convenience and inexpensive food? The irony of meeting in a shiny fast-food restaurant to discuss writing a book on how I dropped 270 pounds was not lost on me. After all, it was eating at places like In-N-Out that got me into heavy trouble in the first place.

Mike and I approached the order counter, and I beckoned for him to go first. I listened to him order a cheeseburger and fries, and that didn't bother me at all. Then I said to the guy in the white cap behind the counter, "I'll have a Double-Double protein burger animal style. And a Diet Coke."

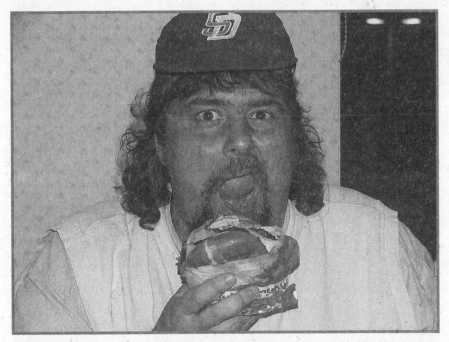

In my bad old days, I loved nothing better than chomping into an In-N-Out 4x4 cheeseburger—as a snack before dinner.

What's a Double-Double protein burger? It's another type of hamburger that you won't find on the In-N-Out menu, but they'll be happy to cook one up for you. Basically, a protein burger is a regular hamburger wrapped in iceberg lettuce—no bun and all protein.

"Animal style" meant that I wanted extra veggies and grilled onions sprinkled on my burger.

If that's what I have to do to maintain my figure these days, then I have no problem eating protein burgers at In-N-Out. Besides, I never want to go back to the old days. These days, the screen saver on my laptop is a full-size picture of me—back when I weighed my heaviest—taking the biggest bite of an In-N-Out 4-by-4. I mean, I was really going for the gusto.

That picture is a daily reminder of how far I've come—and where I never want to go again.

CHAPTER SEVENTEEN
NURTURE WITH LOVE, NOT FOOD

I love being part of a big fat Greek family and being a crazy uncle to my five nephews and nieces. Whenever one of them has a birthday, I give that precious child a day with Uncle Nick to do some toy shopping and share a fun meal in a local restaurant.

After my nephew Josiah turned three recently, I drove him to a Toys "R" Us store in Escondido. "Listen, Little Joey," I said, squatting in the parking lot and getting eye-level with the tykester. "We're going to go into the toy store, and I'll buy anything you want, but I'll buy you only one thing."

"Sure, m'Uncle Nick," he replied with furrowed brow.

I took his hand, and we strode into the store. Immediately, his eyes were captivated by an alluring display of Spiderman figurines atop plastic sleeves filled with M&Ms and Spiderman sugary fruit drinks.

Little Joey yanked on my hand and pulled me toward the endcap display. With his precious little stutter, he said, "Pleeeze, m'Uncle Nick, can I have da Spiderman candy? I want dat," he said, pointing toward Spiderman figurines and M&M candies.

I didn't want him to pick something out in the first thirty seconds of our shopping trip, especially if it was candy! "Joey, don't forget that you can have only one thing, so maybe we better look around the store and see if there is anything else you might want."

"I want dat, I want dat," he said with increasing urgency.

"Why do you want that, Joey?"

"Spiderman on television, m'Uncle Nick."

And it hit me. My little nephew had fallen prey to a strategic marketing campaign aimed at children.

Fortunately, I got Joey to hold off on choosing the Spiderman candy until we could walk down a few aisles. For the next forty-five minutes, he pointed at various toys, and I reached for the box and gave him a closer look. Anything related to Spiderman captured his interest, so it was with some relief when he selected an eighteen-inch Spiderman action figure instead of the Spiderman candy.

I patted myself on the back for successfully distracting him from choosing the junk food. Now it was time for Part B of our adventure— lunch.

"Where would you like to go eat?" I asked Joey.

"M'Uncle Nick, I want McDonald's."

"McDonald's? How about we go for Greek food?"

"No, m'Uncle Nick, I want McDonald's."

"Joey, why do you want to go to McDonalds?"

"McDonald's has Happy Meal. I want McDonald's toy."

Although I was careful not to reveal the boiling anger swelling inside me, I was peeved that my own flesh-and-blood nephew had been victimized by a food marketing campaign that undermines parental authority and fuels the rising ranks of childhood obesity. Joey, an innocent preschooler, was another casualty in the bombardment of food-related advertising. Every time his eyes were glued to Nickelodeon, his impressionable mind soaked up cross-promotional product tie-ins like a sponge. I'm talking about SpongeBob SquarePants Popsicles, Keebler's Scooby Doo cookies, and Incredible Hulk Oreos, to name a few. It's all part of an effort to entice kids like Joey to eat foods high in fat, low in nutrients, and rich in chocolate.

The money spent on marketing fast food, snacks, and beverages to children has doubled in the last ten years. In 2002, big food makers like McDonald's, Pepsico, and Kraft Foods threw $15 billion into Saturday-morning television, cable channels like Nickelodeon and the Cartoon Network, movie tie-ins, video games, Internet Web sites and banner ads, and even in-school marketing to set the hook.

You have to admit the fishing has been pretty good. In 1977, kids ate one in ten meals at a fast-food restaurant. By 1996, that number had jumped to one in three meals, and I don't doubt for one minute that it's higher today. A recent study by the Judge Baker Children's Center in Boston revealed that one in three visits to fast-food restaurants was attributable to the "nag factor"—children begging their parents and wearing them down to take them to a fast-food restaurant. Unfortunately, these children are too young to realize that they are forming eating habits that will set them on the path to obesity.

UNDER SIEGE

From Captain Crunch cereal to Oscar Meyer Lunchables packed with unhealthy fat, and from the Colonel to Ronald McDonald, our children are under siege. Little Joey was swept up by advertising that sends the wrong message: If you eat this food, it will make you happy, cool, and maybe even give you friends.

The Center for Science in the Public Interest recently estimated that only 2 percent of American children eat a diet consistent with the U.S. Department of Agriculture recommendations. The remaining 98 percent of children consume too much fat, sugar, and salt in their food. Small wonder we're raising a nation of couch potato chips. (Chip off the old block, get it?) The Centers for Disease Control predicts that one out of three children born in 2000 will eventually develop type 2 diabetes because they are obese. Some demographers are worried that Joey's generation could be the first to live *fewer* years than today's life expectancy, which is 72.5 years for men and 78.9 years for women, according to the National Center for Health Statistics.

Childhood obesity puts youngsters at risk for multiple medical syndromes. Elevated insulin levels, leading to diabetes, is just one of them. High cholesterol (leading to eventual heart disease), joint stress (leading to eventual degenerative arthritis), and fatty liver disease (leading to liver failure) are among the strong possibilities. Many of these conditions take years to present themselves, but the disease process starts early in life. Obese children are also at much higher risk for developing emotional problems including a negative self-image, and being the victims of hurtful discrimination.

The rising ranks of childhood obesity are finally setting off alarm bells because their numbers have *tripled* since 1980. According to the

Centers for Disease Control and Prevention, 15 percent of children ages six to nineteen are severely overweight, prompting Rick Reilly, the *Sports Illustrated* columnist, to write: "Is your Little Leaguer so fat his blood type is Chee-tos? Do the other kids wait for your Cub Scout to jump in the pool so they can ride the wave? Is it difficult for your six-year-old to play Hide and Seek anymore? *I see you, Amber! At both ends of the Buick!*"

We laugh, but what's sobering is the fact that the biggest growth in obese ranks is among children. "Generation Y is turning into Generation XL," said U.S. Surgeon General Richard H. Carmona.

The following revelation may surprise you, but I was not an obese kid when I grew up. I spent most of my childhood in Greece, where my parents had a household rule that is hard for many of my current friends to comprehend: We had no TV set. There was no such thing as TV time.

My childhood was spent chasing soccer balls, swimming in the Mediterranean, riding bikes, going on exploratory hikes with my brothers through the foothills of Athens, and spending hour after hour running around. That's not what kids do today after school. Within minutes after stepping off the school bus (no exercise there), they plop down in front of the TV set with bowls of chocolate ice cream on their laps.

I feel sorry for today's kids. When Mom and Dad work outside the home, latchkey kids are told to stay inside the house because it's safe. There isn't much to do except watch TV, play video games, and snack on Snackwells. They aren't getting enough exercise at school, either: School districts, faced with shrinking budgets and demands to bring up standardized test scores, are dropping gym classes to save money.

PE classes, once mandatory, are now an elective in many school districts across the nation, so fewer kids are involved in school-coordinated physical activity.

It breaks my heart to see the Chee-tos generation in my examination room. Child after child, bulging at the seams, is weighed down with fat and lowered expectations of their futures. These children are eating way too many calories way too early in life. Instead of riding bikes or running around the neighborhood after school, they live a sedentary lifestyle filled with TV, video games, and chatting with their friends on the Internet. Teens are hooked on their cell phones, yakking between classes, making calls after school, and tapping out text messages. The only limbs they exercise are at the end of their arms—the thumbs, fingers, and wrists.

If you were sitting in my examination room today, I would share the following action points with you and your child. Please receive them in the spirit they are offered, which is humility. Nonetheless, please know that there is a righteous anger burning within me because I don't want your children growing up with schoolyard taunting and teasing because they're fat. I'm sure it's your ultimate desire, as parents, to see them thrive and excel while living the healthiest life possible.

Point #1: Love and accept your children as they are.

You must affirm and confirm your children, no matter what their weight may be. Never be critical or hostile about their weight, or you will crush their tender spirits. Their physical appearance is not the issue. How they look should be irrelevant to you. Your desire is for them to live long, healthy, and productive lives.

Point #2: Remember that you're the parent, so your children's health is your responsibility.

Allow me to put on my Dr. Laura hat for a moment and speak a little tough love. Listen, kids are your responsibility. You are your kid's mom, your kid's dad. Don't let Saturday morning cartoons have more influence over your children than you do. Don't let them watch TV! You are probably unaware of this, but there's a battle going on for your children's hearts and attention, and the other side can call on tremendous resources. It would be great if someone were out there aggressively marketing vegetables and fruit, but that's not happening. What is getting marketed is sugar and fat in toxic concentrations.

The big food companies will tell you their foods have a place in a balanced diet, which prompts me to say, "Show me the darn balance." I don't see any balance in the way kids eat today. Kids, if left to their own devices, would tug at you like Little Joey to take them to McDonald's for lunch *and* dinner every day. Why should you relinquish the parental authority to establish appropriate and healthy eating behaviors to a faceless conglomerate that wants to feed your children unhealthy food?

I understand that it's unrealistic not to have a TV in the home. But what's wrong with setting some limits when TV can be watched and video games can be played? When my parents finally broke down and purchased a TV in my teen years, my father made a hard-and-fast rule: We could watch TV for only one hour a day, and for every hour of TV we watched, we had to read for two hours.

Maybe the reading part would be over the top these days, but I think one hour of TV—after dinner—is more than enough. If your children are not allowed to watch TV or play video games after school, they will be forced to find something else to do. The first week or two will be rough on everyone as the whine factor cranks up to high-pitch volumes. Get them involved in soccer leagues. Buy them bikes. Take them swimming. Go for after-dinner walks together. Whatever you do, though, don't let them go to their friends' house unless those parents aren't allowing their kids to watch TV and play video games. Otherwise, your kids will watch TV or play Nintendo games over there.

Whenever I suggest severely limiting the TV in my examination room, you should see the look of incredulous disbelief in the faces of the parents. *Are you joking? Do you realize how many programs there are for my kid to watch? I can't afford a babysitter.*

I won't budge in this advice because it's the only way to break the stranglehold that food advertising has on kids and get them moving their bodies. A congressional ban of fast-food advertising will never happen, so it's up to you to rein in the electronic images coming into your home.

Point #3: Be able to advise, "Do as I say, and as I have done."

I know for years, I used to say one thing and do another. My credibility as a doctor took a hit all those years, and I don't want that to happen to you. That's why your declarations that you're going to stay away from junk food may fall on deaf ears if you're constantly relenting "just this once." Kids stop listening when you say one thing and do another.

Furthermore, you may have to walk the talk by getting your own derriere in shape first. If the kids are old enough, take them to the gym with you. If you join a fitness emporium like an LA Fitness or a YMCA, the children can swim, play basketball or racquetball, or ride stationary bikes. After-dinner family walks in the warm twilight promote good health *and* healthy interpersonal relationships. Becoming healthier should be a family event, so don't single out your heavy children in the process.

Point #4: *Fill the fridge and the cupboards with the right stuff.*

Kids have a way of eating what's inside the refrigerator and the cupboards. So what are you filling your shopping carts with? Treats wrapped in plastic? Aluminum cans filled with sugary sodas? Cartons of artery-clogging ice cream? Frozen pizzas?

I'm not suggesting that you shop at a health food store or fill the refrigerator with brussels sprouts and tofu. But having a wide assortment of fruits available—apples, tangerines, and bananas—and breads made with whole wheat flour can pull the kids off the Twinkie-and-Ding-Dong treadmill. Consider peeling and slicing various kinds of fruit, thereby making a healthy snack readily available and convenient to eat. Make your home a no-soda zone.

Kids are born to snack, but snacking on sweets an hour before dinner suppresses their appetites. By the time everyone gathers for supper, they're not hungry—and your homemade meat loaf won't be desirable to them. Neither will your cooked vegetables. Two hours later, however, they're hungry again, and they're sneaking Oreos by the handful. You can see how it's a vicious circle.

Kids are just like adults—food tastes better when they're hungry, so if they're *starved* before mealtime, feed them something healthy like carrot sticks or a sliced apple. Snacks should be snacks—not mid-afternoon desserts. If you give them access to eat anything they want before dinner, you'll get frustrated if they don't eat something that took you forty-five minutes to prepare.

And that's not good for you or for them.

Point #5: Replace fast-food forays with home-cooked meals.
I'm not suggesting that you and your family abstain from fast food for
the rest of your lives. I see nothing wrong with going to McDonald's
or Jack in the Box on occasion. By occasion, I mean one meal a week.

Nonetheless, I realize that many young families don't go to Burger
King—they just end up there. You know the drill: it's 6 p.m., the kids'
soccer practice is over, there's nothing in the fridge, you worked all
day, and you're too tired to cook. So you and the family succumb to
the siren call of fast food.

I have just the solution for you, and it's one my mother practiced
for many years: Always have leftovers on hand. Mom never knew
when company would drop in at our home, so she always cooked a
huge main dish that we could get two or three meals out of. Having
leftovers in the fridge is the perfect answer for those evenings when
you're too tired to cook, haven't shopped, or have run out of time.
Heat up some leftovers in a pan with olive oil or butter, set out some
salad, and you're eating in the same amount of time it would take to
pass through the drive-thru lane. Besides, I think leftovers are often
tastier the second time around.

You should also keep a stash of ready-to-go food in the freezer. For
instance, you can brown ten pounds of ground turkey with onions
and then package it in one-pound freezer bags. The same idea works
with chicken breasts. Pop those bags in the microwave, and within
minutes you have the fixings for a meal on the go: chicken and wild
rice, hamburger spaghetti, chicken fajitas, sloppy joes, and so forth.
Don't overlook the Crock-Pot, either. Brown some meat in the morning, dice up some fresh vegetables, add chicken broth and water, and
you'll have a delicious meal that evening.

Finally, let me make a pitch for the value of eating dinner together. I know the concept of family fellowship is ingrained in me because I grew up with *koinonia*, but there's much to be said for the value of both generations sitting down and sharing what happened during the day. Dinnertime is usually the only time that busy families can slow down and share a meal and their lives together You will have to *work* at making this happen, and once you sit down, don't be in a hurry for the meal to finish.

Dinner meals promote family togetherness, foster communication, and have a remarkable impact on children. A study published in the *American Psychological Society* newsletter revealed that teenagers who eat with their parents five times or more a week were less likely to do drugs or be depressed and more likely to be motivated students.

Another important point about teens: They eat better when Mom (or Dad) is cooking for them. Left alone on a Saturday night, they would heat up a frozen pizza, which is nothing more than a slab of cardboard topped with weak tomato sauce. Look at cooking for your teens as an antidote to the fast-food culture in which they are growing up. Asking them to help out with meal preparation will give them an appreciation for different foods and for the effort it takes to serve healthy, delicious meals. Every time you serve your children a well-balanced, home-cooked meal, you reverse the odometer of obesity.

Point #6: Remember that food is nutrition—not an incentive program, a form of punishment, a reward for doing something good, or a way of showing love.

My parents rewarded me with ice cream for finishing my homework. They took food away when they disciplined me. They also turned a blind eye, while still entertaining friends at the dinner table, while I helped myself to another serving of pasta with feta and Parmesan cheese.

I understand, even though I don't have kids yet, that there isn't a parent alive who hasn't "treated" their children at Baskin-Robbins. That's why it's called a treat. If a treat is small and reserved for an occasion, I have no problem with that. It's just that I have a problem with parents who pull into the Dunkin' Donuts parking lot every day they drive their children to school.

Point #7: Keep your kids in PE classes.

The lack of physical activity is a significant contributor to obesity, and those who do exercise do better in the classroom. Every medical organization I've been a part of recommends daily PE from kindergarten through the senior year of high school.

School boards around the country are cutting PE classes to balance their budgets. Some are lowering their PE requirements to graduate from high school to one or two years, or students can skip gym class if they're in band or cheerleading.

No matter what shape your children are in, keep them in PE, where they're doing calisthenics, push-ups, running the mile, and generally breaking a sweat. PE classes aren't *the* answer to childhood obesity, but they are certainly an integral part of a healthy lifestyle.

What isn't healthy these days is the way soft-drink companies and fast-food chains have infiltrated school campuses with vending machines dispensing sodas and cafeterias serving up "Pizza Hut Wednesdays" and "Taco Bell Fridays." In 1990, only 2 percent of American school districts included Pizza Hut or Taco Bell food as part of their school-based nutritional programs. In 2000, that number moved up to 20 percent. These exclusive contracts between the fast-food companies and the schools feel like dollars falling out of the sky to pragmatic school district officials, whose budgets have been squeezed by state legislatures and an apathetic citizenry that rarely votes to approve much-needed school bonds. The motivation behind the sweet deals is that a captive audience—your kids—will become "brand loyal" consumers who will stay with the brand their entire lifetimes.

When I graduated from high school, the sweetest thing you could buy in the cafeteria was Hawaiian Punch. Today, the kids arrive in the morning and buy breakfast from a vending machine: Doritos and Cherry Coke or Skittles and Mountain Dew. For lunch, it's Pepsi, Pizza Hut pepperoni pizza, and a Mars candy bar. No wonder some of the kids have acne and weight problems. All day long, it's sugar, sugar, sugar and fat, fat, fat.

I forgot to mention the caffeine. Drinks such as Mountain Dew, Surge, Josta, and Jolt deliver a caffeine punch—92 milligrams per twenty-ounce drink, or the equivalent of a five-ounce cup of brewed coffee. Caffeine causes nervousness, irritability, restlessness and fidgetiness, which means that teachers must contend with caffeine-hopping kids in the period immediately following the lunch bell.

Parents, I encourage you to feed your children a nutritious breakfast before school and pack a sack lunch with a sandwich made from whole wheat bread, a piece of fruit, and a "sweet" like some dates or other dried fruit. The other thing is to keep your eyes open. Did you know that Krispy Kreme has a nationwide program offering kids one doughnut for each A on their report cards? Not only is that ploy using food as a reward, but it's using unhealthy food, and that's not good for your children's health.

IF YOUR CHILD IS OBESE . . .

Then you've got to do something about it. You're the parent, right? I mean, I would love to see a company step up to the plate and invent a treadmill or a stationary bike that doesn't let the TV come on until the person is walking or pedaling fast enough, but that hasn't happened yet.

If your child is obese (more than fifty pounds over his weight chart), you don't have any time to lose because childhood pounds— once puberty kicks in—are very tough to lose. In addition, the teen brain "wires" the adult brain. Patterns of thought and behavior established in adolescence are adopted as "default settings" the rest of your children's lives, according to Duke University biological research psychologist Aaron White. Teens who don't exercise are unlikely to pick up that habit after age twenty, and choices about overeating are difficult to overcome.

Now is the time for action. You can apply the foundational principles of the Seven Pillars to your children. Be encouraging as you help them see the way they are so they can change the way they look. Since you're doing the cooking, you can slash their calories, but it's up to them to eat the right amount of the right foods when they're out of the house. We've established ways to get them exercising more than their thumbs and forefingers, and finally, as their parent, you can be by their side so they don't have to travel alone.

In planning a radical sabbatical, I could recommend a summer "weight-loss" camp. For example, here in San Diego we have Camp La Jolla, a two-month program where students board at my old stomping grounds—the University of California of San Diego (UCSD). Camp La Jolla bills itself as a weight-loss, fitness, and health vacation camp at the beach where kids discover new friends, improve their health, and gain great self-esteem, while losing weight, too.

I think something like a Camp La Jolla would be a great "radical sabbatical" for young people to change the way they see before they change the way they look. There are dozens of these weight-loss camps around the country, and I would check them out.

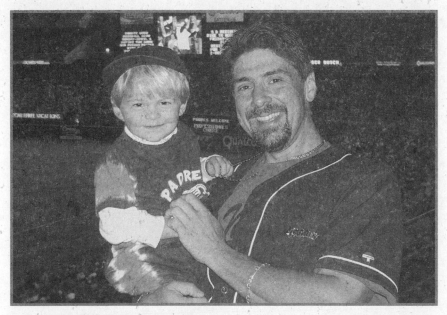

It's a treat to attend Opening Day baseball games, as I did with my nephew Joey in April 2003.

Meanwhile, I think there are some interim steps you can take *today* to help fulfill the Seven Pillars. You can:

- Stop frequenting fast-food restaurants.
- Cook meals from scratch.
- Have healthy snacks in the house.
- Make sure your children are getting thirty to ninety minutes

of exercise every day.

- Limit TV time.
- Join a fitness club.
- Plan healthy vacations, like skiing, hiking, mountain bike riding, swimming, and water-skiing.

Mom, Dad, I know how difficult your assignment is because I've worked with parents who wanted to turn their children's lives around. But your sustained effort to see this through will affect not only your children's lives, but also the lives of your children's children.

There's a lot at stake here. Step up to the plate and do the right thing for those you love the most.

CHAPTER EIGHTEEN

HEIGH-HO, HEIGH-HO, IT'S UNDER THE KNIFE WE GO

One of my favorite things about medicine is the relationship I can develop with my patients over the course of time. I put a lot of energy into my bedside manner, and I strongly believe that my empathetic demeanor helps sick people get back on the road to recovery.

My heart always goes out to morbidly obese patients hospitalized for complications relating to their unhealthy condition—severe diabetes, heart failure, and crippling joint disease, just to name a few. I know that but for the grace of God, I could be lying in the same bed, wondering if my days were numbered as well. Inevitably, I pull up a chair and take extra time to visit with these hurting folks. When I sense they need a boost of encouragement, I reach into my leather-bound planner and show them a picture of me wedged into a stadium seat at a San Diego Padre game.

"Do you recognize that person?" I ask.

"No, who is he?" is the response I generally hear, but that's probably because I was wearing curly, shoulder-length hair atop a torso brimming with 467 pounds.

"That was me four years ago," I say.

The responses range from "No way" to "I don't believe you." After the initial shock and hyperventilation pass, they always say, "How did the surgery go?"

How did the surgery go?

That's the nearly universal reaction I receive when I show overweight patients the "before" photos. They automatically assume that the only way I could have shed so much weight was by having some sort of gastric bypass operation, or what the media calls "stomach stapling" surgery.

I find that reaction understandable but bothersome since these people—who don't bear any ill will toward me—figure that anyone who loses seventy-five, one hundred, or two hundred pounds of weight did so only by going under the knife. That supposition is largely based on the waves of publicity given to celebrities who have experienced dramatic weight loss from gastric bypass surgery. I'm thinking of Al Roker, the *Today Show* weatherman; Carnie Wilson, the talented singer with Wilson Phillips; and Sharon Osbourne, the wife of Ozzy Osbourne and a central character of the MTV reality show *The Osbournes.*

I would be the first to agree that the surgical results have been stunning for this trio of telegenic personalities. Al, who lost more than one hundred pounds after submitting to gastric bypass surgery, is treated like a rock star when he steps outside the NBC studio in Rockefeller Center and mingles with the fans during his weather segment. Carnie, the daughter of Beach Boys legend Brian Wilson, *is* a rock star, and she ballooned beyond three hundred pounds as her career took off. For years, however, she struggled to cope with depression and soaring success until she underwent gastric bypass surgery. She looks marvelous today. Sharon Osbourne is an engaging Brit *married* to a rock star. She told *Us* magazine that she'd weigh five hundred pounds and push herself around in a wheelchair if she hadn't had her stomach "banded." Like me, she had to beat cancer before turning her attention to her dirigible-like weight. Her weight dropped from 224 pounds to around 130 pounds.

I'm happy that these celebrities have become spokespersons for gastric bypass surgery, which is becoming more popular by the minute. For a certain segment of the obese population, gastric bypass is a valid option and has helped hundreds of thousands of formerly heavy people regain some normalcy to their lives, which is great to see. My joy is tempered, however, by the serious health risks associated with this type of surgery, and these risks should be carefully considered before submitting to a major surgical procedure on one of the most delicate areas of the body—the digestive system.

THE EXPLOSION IN SCALPEL SOLUTIONS

These days, gastric bypass surgery is the hot trend in weight-loss circles. Obese people are flocking to the extra-wide operating tables in surgery bays around the country and saying, "Sew up my stomach!"

The number of bypass operations exploded from 23,100 in 1997 to more than 100,000 in 2003, according to the American Society for Bariatric Surgery, a nearly fourfold increase in just six years. Hospitals can't keep up with the demand: At Tufts-New England Medical Center in Boston, doctors cut off the waiting list at five hundred people, saying they needed six months to catch up. You're looking at a twelve- to eighteen-month wait at many hospitals across the country.

Talk about a growth industry. The number of doctors joining the American Society for Bariatric Surgery—the physicians who specialize in this sort of surgery—has also tripled in the last five years, and a national company called Bariatric Treatments Centers recently opened a forty-seven-bed hospital outside Philadelphia just for bypass patients. Other BTCs have opened their doublewide doors in places like Dallas; Grove City, Ohio; Scottsdale, Arizona; and Holland, Michigan. The demand for gastric bypass is clearly outstripping the supply.

So what is gastric bypass surgery? Why is it so popular? In layman's terms, gastric bypass promotes weight loss by surgically restricting food intake and/or interrupting the normal digestive process. What surgeons do is staple the stomach—or bind it with an adjustable band—and create a small pouch big enough to hold two or three ounces of food—a handful of food—before it's passed along to the rest of the digestive tract.

A normal adult stomach can hold three pints of food at one sitting—around twenty-four ounces, which is a large plate of food. When I was in the prime of my eating career, my stomach could hold more than that. I had a world-class gut—a super-duper deluxe model that could probably take in six or seven pints of food. I could eat people under the table, like I did with reckless abandon during the Last Supper.

Clearly, you don't need that large a stomach to survive, but people start eating and they don't know when to stop because they aren't full yet, or they eat beyond their natural sensation of being full. Gastric bypass surgery changes all that by reducing the stomach to *one-tenth* of the size it used to be. It doesn't take a brain surgeon to figure out that you're going to get that "full" feeling very quickly and lose your appetite rapidly. Eat any more, and you become nauseated and want to vomit. *That'll keep you from eating too much.*

Gastric bypass surgery was developed fifty years ago after surgeons unexpectedly discovered that patients having large portions of their stomach or small intestine removed—either for severe stomach ulcers or advanced forms of stomach cancer—universally lost weight after the procedure.

The first record of a surgeon's *intentionally* stapling off the intestines, called an intestinal bypass, is from 1954. This invasive surgery often caused severe complications, however, so other methods of bypassing the stomach were developed over the decades, but doctors still had to make a six-inch gash and open up the belly to get at the stomach. It wasn't until the 1990s when doctors developed laparoscopic surgery techniques that allowed them to insert surgical instruments into the abdomen, along with a tiny camera. These days, the incisions are much smaller, and the lead surgeon watches a TV monitor while he works his instruments inside the gut and performs delicate procedures that were unthinkable a half century ago. Carnie Wilson, who took advantage of this new laparoscopic technology, broadcast her operation over the Internet.

So, who's a candidate for stomach stapling? To qualify for gastric bypass surgery, you must have a body mass index (BMI) of more than 40. For men, this typically means they are at least one hundred pounds overweight, and for women, at least eighty pounds beyond their healthy weight range. An interesting side note: 80 percent of the people in our country with BMIs of 40 or more are women of child-bearing age. The surgery is also indicated for patients with a BMI of 35 or higher if other major weight-related complications exist, such as sleep apnea, arthritis, or heart disease. Health insurance companies use these criteria to determine eligibility for coverage.

Gastric bypass surgery is generally reserved for morbidly obese individuals who have made numerous unsuccessful attempts at losing weight through traditional methods—going on diets, changing eating patterns, working with nutritionists, and increasing physical activity. It's supposed to be the treatment of last resort, but that's not how it's currently being marketed or perceived by the public. I've heard of surgeons promoting gastric bypass surgery for those with only forty or fifty pounds to lose. That's not a healthy or appropriate choice for patients with that amount of excess weight.

The surgery is not cheap. You better have good health insurance because the procedure costs around $25,000. Complications drive up the price. Since many health plans do not cover the full amount, you could be responsible for 20 percent, which means you could have out-of-pocket expenses of $5,000. If you're poor or uninsured, as most of my patients are, you can forget about gastric bypass surgery. In many states, the overburdened public health system doesn't pay for this sort of procedure. Medi-Cal patients in my home state can face a twelve-year wait for bariatric surgery.

THE OPTIONS

What hasn't sunk in for many considering gastric bypass is that you get a free ride only for the first year. In other words, it takes your body about a year to recover from the surgery and to assimilate the limitations imposed by the surgeon's knife. Initially, the weight drops off effortlessly, but after a while your body compensates for the changes in your anatomy. Suddenly, you stop losing weight. If you fail to practice the same good eating and exercise habits that accompany every other diet regimen, you will regain some of the weight lost. The truth is that the only way to lose weight and keep it off is to take in fewer calories than you expend, as I've been saying all along. *It's calories in and calories out . . .* there are no shortcuts to successful weight management!

Gastric bypass surgery is not a shortcut to weight loss, nor should it be viewed that way. It should be reserved for men and women who have struggled with long-term obesity and have carefully studied the pros and cons of this procedure. I realize that gastric bypass may be your last chance at leading a "normal" life, and that's how I prefer to view this surgery—as a procedure for those in their eighth or ninth innings of active life, people who have exhausted every other avenue toward weight loss.

Basically, you have four different options when it comes to gastric bypass surgery. With most of the surgical variations, a skilled surgeon creates a small pouch at the top of the stomach by using a band or staples (which is why it's sometimes called "stomach stapling"). At the lower end of this newly fashioned pouch, a small opening is made, which slows the movement of food considerably. This is another reason why a person has that "full feeling" so quickly after eating something. If you eat too much or too fast, you feel ill immediately. Here are the specific options for those considering some form of gastric bypass surgery:

Adjustable Banded Gastroplasty, or ABG

The surgeon places an adjustable gastric band laparoscopically around the upper stomach. The band squeezes the stomach, creating a small pouch for food to enter and a narrow passage out into the remaining portion of the stomach. If you do not lose the desired weight, the surgeon can always go back in and cinch up the adjustable band to change the size of the passage through which ingested food must pass through. This restricts further the amount of food that one can tolerate eating at any one time.

Pros: The least invasive surgery, with a minimal change of normal anatomy.

Cons: High risk of vomiting, risk of band slippage, pouch stretching, and less successful than more invasive options.

Vertical Banded Gastroplasty, or VBG

Similar to an ABG, the Vertical Banded Gastroplasty also creates a small pouch in the upper stomach with a narrow outlet but does so by using both a band and staples.

Pros: Less invasive than bypass procedures.

Cons: Potential for wearing away of the band or the breakdown of the staple line, less successful than more invasive options, high risk of vomiting, and pouch stretching.

Roux-en-Y Gastric Bypass (RYGB)

The RYGB is considered to be the most common and successful form of gastric bypass surgery. Besides creating a small pouch, a Y-shaped section of the small intestine—called the "Roux limb"—is brought up and attached to the pouch. Food, therefore, bypasses the lower stomach completely plus the first portion of the small intestine. Not only does the patient feel full after eating a small amount, but part of the intestinal tract, where calories and nutrients are absorbed, is bypassed.

This can be good if you're looking to reduce caloric intake, but this can be bad because your body is missing out on important nutrients. That's why doctors recommend that patients take vitamins and nutritional supplements such as iron and calcium for the rest of their lives.

The Roux-en-Y is the surgery of choice for most bariatric surgeons in the U.S., who call it the single most successful procedure for excess weight loss and long-term weight control. With intensive counseling, support, and nutrition education, proponents claim a long-term success rate of nearly 90 percent. Success is defined as maintaining a weight loss of 50 percent or more of one's excess weight for up to ten years. For instance, someone who weighed 300 pounds (with an ideal body weight of 160 pounds) would be considered successful if he or she continued to weigh 230 pounds or less after the surgery.

Pros: Produces more weight loss than less invasive surgeries and makes it more likely that patients will reverse health complications related to obesity.

Cons: Higher risk for nutritional deficiencies, surgical complications, waves of nausea and light-headedness.

Bilio Pancreatic Diversion Technique, or BPD

This is the most radical and complicated treatment since part of the stomach is actually removed. The small pouch that remains is connected to the final portion of the small intestine. This means a much larger portion of the small intestine is completely bypassed, which dramatically reduces caloric absorption. Though not employed very often, proponents say that the Bilio Pancreatic Diversion requires *less* effort on part of the patients to make it work for them.

You have to stop eating fatty foods with the BPD. If you don't, you and your family members will be on the receiving end of massive amounts of flatulence. You'll also be running to the toilet with constant diarrhea.

Pros: You're nearly guaranteed to experience massive weight loss.

Cons: Very high risk of nutritional deficiency, more likely to experience surgical side effects, and flatulence.

New Surgical Frontiers

You should be aware that bariatric doctors are working on an implanted gastric stimulator that fools the body into feeling full, which would be an alternative to undergoing digestive tract surgery. Called a "stomach pacemaker," doctors implant an electrical pulse generator under the skin in the abdomen near the stomach's major nerves. Electrical stimulation dulls the appetite, giving people that icky too full feeling. The stomach pacemaker is currently on the market in Europe, though the Food and Drug Administration (FDA) has not yet approved it. Many doctors believe that because the implanting of the pacemaker is not too invasive and is considered minor surgery, this kind of procedure could prove to be an effective alternative to the popular gastric bypass surgery.

A VOICE IN THE GRANDSTANDS

Here's where I come down on gastric bypass surgery, and I'm going to tell you by using a word picture. Let's pretend that you're the manager of a major-league baseball team. You've had a rough start to the game—every pitcher you send to the mound gets shelled, and now you're down to one pitcher in your bullpen. Fortunately for your side, your hitters are having a big night, so the game is tied at 14–14 in the fifth inning.

Your next-to-last pitcher keeps giving up hits, but you hope he can weather the storm. Or do you bring in your last pitcher to put out the fire, even though it's only the fifth inning? But if you do that, your last pitcher has to keep hurling the rest of the game.

Stomach stapling surgery is the same thing. In my mind, it's your last shot—your last pitcher on the roster. What happens if gastric bypass doesn't work? That happens, you know. Up to 20 percent of all patients need follow-up surgery to correct a complication such as the breakdown of the band, hernias in the abdominal wall, and stretched-out pouches. As with any major surgery, there are significant health risks associated with it. Fortunately, as the techniques improve, the adverse side effects are becoming less common, but they are still there.

One side effect is that food bypasses certain key parts of the small intestine, and this interferes with the absorption of essential nutrients. Nutritional deficiencies can lead to anemia, osteoporosis, and other bone diseases. There is also the risk of something called "dumping syndrome," which is an uncomfortable wave of nausea and weakness, along with sweating and a feeling of light-headedness. Oh, and don't forget the potential for explosive diarrhea.

Death is the ultimate complication. The chances of your dying from the surgery are rather high in my book—around one in two hundred, maybe a little less, maybe a little more, depending on whose stats you see. The risk of dying is dependent on the kind of surgery, the patient's medical condition at the time of surgery, and complications that crop up during surgery. Still, a mortality rate of between 0.5 and 1 percent is uncomfortably high when you compare the chance of dying from a smallpox vaccination, which is one in a million. Critics were howling when smallpox vaccinations started up in 2003 following the terrorist threat. But isn't it interesting that there isn't a peep of protest when one in two hundred gastric-bypass recipients die from complications following their surgery? There have also been cases of patients dying after binge-eating and rupturing the staples.

MAKING THE WEIGHTY DECISION

I understand why people are willing to take the risk. There's no doubt that significant weight loss improves self-image and self-esteem; no one understands that better than I do. There are many morbidly obese individuals who are totally incapacitated and unable to work. These folks could regain active social lives, take part in physical activities, or even be gainfully employed. Many patients who have type 2 diabetes, primarily related to their obesity, can literally be cured of their illness. Further improvements can occur in cardiac function, blood pressure, and breathing problems like sleep apnea. Ultimately, patients can experience a dramatic improvement in the quality of life.

Nonetheless, I've met and corresponded with too many people who could not stop overeating, despite the presence of a stomach the size of an egg inside their abdomens. One woman melted milk chocolate bars in a coffee cup in her microwave oven and sipped liquefied chocolate all day. Others purée food that wasn't meant to be puréed—Krispy Kremes, Twinkies, and birthday cakes. Another woman confessed to me that she ground up pistachio nuts and ate them all afternoon. Although these folks couldn't eat as much, they were constantly grazing—a nonstop, slow, consistent nibbling of food. In each case they regained all the weight they had lost.

Even more disturbing to me is that some physicians are recommending that children as young as thirteen undergo gastric bypass surgery. Tufts-New England Medical Center—the hospital with a long waiting list—mailed letters to a thousand pediatricians, saying, in so many words, "Send us your kids." Their rationale: Let's surgically intervene now before these fat kids develop some real problems, like diabetes, joint damage, and heart disease.

Excuse me, but the thought of stomach stapling a seventh grader strikes me as misguided at best and bordering on medical malpractice at worst. This is a lifelong decision with lifelong implications. Again, I return to my baseball analogy: Performing a gastric bypass operation on a minor is like using your last pitcher in the second inning. Who is left in the bull pen? Answer: No one.

I understand that gastric bypass surgery may be a necessity for some. Many who've struggled with obesity all their lives have truly exhausted their options, and they are suffering from serious complications of severe obesity. If, in partnership with their physicians, they have thoughtfully worked through the process and concluded that surgery is truly their option of last resort, they should proceed without hesitation.

NO EASY ANSWERS

Nonetheless, I must say that I'm concerned with all this momentum building toward surgical intervention, what with the influence of celebrities like Al Roker and Sharon Osbourne and a growing medical industry aggressively marketing it. I received pressure to undergo gastric bypass surgery as well from my colleagues. I still haven't forgotten the time a few years ago when another physician caught me in the hallway and said, "Hey, Big Nick, have you thought about having surgery when you're ready to do something about that weight?"

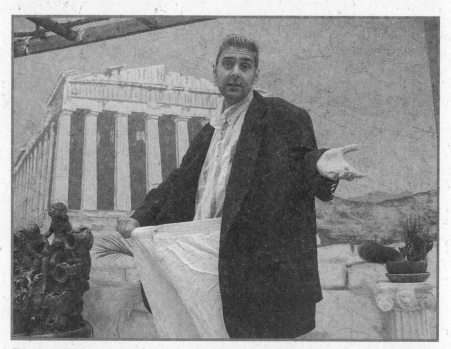

This picture was taken shortly after my "makeover" in November 2001, when I went from looking like an unemployed NFL lineman to a member of a boy band.

I may be a voice in the wilderness, the only person sitting in a vast stadium, but I am a visible reminder that dramatic change is possible *without* surgery. Sure, I know that the chips are stacked against us. I know that 90 percent of people who lose weight put it right back on again. The point I want to get across is that obesity is a complicated issue with no easy answers, and stomach stapling should be the *last-resort* option. Even for those who have the surgery, it still comes back to eating the right amount of the right food in the right way, adding exercise to their lifestyle, and changing the way they see so that they can change the way they look.

The bottom line remains the same. Don't bring in your last pitcher until it's absolutely necessary and all else has failed. Please!

CHAPTER NINETEEN
THE LAST COURSE

The toughest letter I ever wrote was that of April 1, 2000, when I gave notice to the Escondido Community Health Center that I would be resigning as medical director effective April 1, 2001.

"My motivation for this 'break' is really a simple one—my health," I wrote. "Unfortunately, with the pace of life and scope of involvements, mixed with a lack of discipline, I have neglected a key part of my being."

This was a nice way of saying, *I've let myself go for years and became a Goodyear blimp. Now I have to do something about it.*

My resignation letter sent shock waves throughout the local community. "Nick, you have really lost it," one friend told me. "You mean to tell me that you're leaving work and going to baseball games to lose weight? You're one sick puppy."

Faced with this barrage of criticism, self-doubts surfaced within me.

Maybe I was doing something too drastic. Maybe I hadn't thought things through. Maybe I wasn't thinking clearly. Several weeks later, in May 2000, I was seriously questioning my decision. Maybe I had acted too hastily. Maybe things weren't *that* bad.

That was my thinking on the day I received a page from home. Like every doctor, I have an electronic leash attached to my belt—a pager. Since I received dozens of calls a day, I thought up a special code for my family. For a routine call, they tapped in their phone number. If they needed to talk to me in the next five or ten minutes, they tapped in 777 after their phone number. If it was an emergency, they were to tap in a 9-1-1 tag after the phone number.

I remember giving one of my brothers a piece of my mind the time he dialed 911 to make sure I stopped by the store to pick up some feta cheese. So when I received a 911 page on a Friday afternoon in May, I wasn't expecting to hear the frantic screaming of my mother on the line. "Nicky, Dad was weeding the garden and collapsed to the ground!" she cried out with great fear in her voice. "I already called 911, but please come quickly. I don't want him to die!"

"I'll be right there!"

I drove like a crazy man. By the time I arrived home ten minutes later, four paramedics were preparing him for transport to Palomar Medical Center.

I kneeled by his side in the backyard. "Dad, are you okay?" I asked.

He could barely respond. He clutched his chest and moaned, and I felt helpless. I never expected to see my father stricken by a heart attack. Dad had never smoked a cigarette in his adult life, and he had never been treated for high blood pressure or diabetes. Sure, he was forty pounds overweight, but he was an active sixty-six-year-old who wasn't afraid to get his hands dirty in his garden. His little sin was a weakness for roasted lamb, hard-shell bread, and olives.

I could tell just by looking at Dad that he was barely hanging on to life. The paramedics rushed him to the hospital, where an angiogram revealed that he had 95 percent blockage of the main coronary artery. Doctors stabilized him until an operation several days later when he underwent successful quintuple bypass surgery.

Dad was granted a new lease on life, but his heart attack put to rest any lingering doubts regarding my decision to take a sabbatical and go on a weight-loss journey. What I was planning to do had become a matter of life and death. Now I *had* to go.

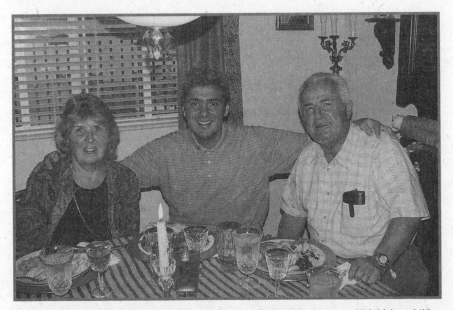

Mom and Dad have loved me unconditionally all my life, through the proverbial thick and thin, and for that I owe them a debt of gratitude that can never be repaid.

If you can be classified as obese or beyond, you have a life-and-death decision to make. So what are you going to do? Are you going to put down this book and say, *You know, Dr. Nick, you have a great story, and I really should do something about my weight some day, but . . . ?*

If I hadn't done something, I wouldn't have gone from shame to determination and from despair to hope. If I hadn't done something, I wouldn't have gone from a size 60 waist to a size 36. If I hadn't done something, I would still be worrying where I would sit in a restaurant or on a passenger jet. If I hadn't done something, I would be receiving stares of disapproval everywhere I went in public.

What happened to me was a big fat Greek miracle. It was as though I'd been born again and given back my life. There's no other way to explain it, except to say that what happened to me happened by the grace of God.

Please consider your future. Do something before it's too late. Don't wait until tomorrow. You can change the way you see so you can change the way you look. I know you can plan a radical sabbatical and find an accountability partner.

Hopefully, I've inspired you with my story and given you plenty of ideas about how you can lose weight once and for all.

So, what are you going to do about it?

EPILOGUE

You might have noticed that I dedicated this book to "my Despina."

If you're wondering who—or what—Despina is, she is the love of my life. She is my sunshine and the air I breathe, and she also goes by Mrs. Despina Yphantides.

On May 1, 2004, in my hometown of Escondido before our extended families, Despina Christopoulos became my lawfully wedded wife, to have and to hold from this day forward, for better or worse, for richer or poorer, in sickness and in health, to love and to cherish until death do us part.

As you would expect, we had our own big fat Greek wedding. We were tempted to invite fifteen hundred of our closest friends to join us for a blowout celebration because so many friends and patients had said over the years, "Dr. Nick, when you get hitched, you've got to invite me . . ." We decided, however, to keep our wedding an intimate, family-centered event.

I met Despina in the midst of writing this book during the fall of 2003. Talk about distractions. Despina—"Debi" to her American friends—is a Greek-American like me whose family roots can be traced back to New Jersey, where I originally grew up. We were born in the same hospital and grew up a half mile away from each other in Bergen County, although we never knew each other.

A cousin back in New Jersey, Gail Malatesta, was the family member who tried to set me up with Despina. Many relatives like Gail and well-meaning friends had long been trying to "fix" me up with someone, but I had resisted any matchmaking efforts. This is the twenty-first century, after all.

My dad happened to call Gail in early October 2003 to check on how things were going with her mother—Dad's sister—in Greece. During the conversation, Gail, frustrated with my lack of response to her efforts, suggested that my father intervene. She insisted that Despina would be a wonderful match, and besides, she lived in nearby Dana Point, a Southern California coastal community less than an hour from Escondido.

Dad, who is a throwback, took matters into his own hands to meet this Despina. I happened to be out of town for a week on a sixty-mile hike in the High Sierra. Dad boldly called her and introduced himself, and they agreed to meet that afternoon for a Sunday evening service at Saddleback Church in Lake Forest, which Despina attended. Afterward, my father invited her out for a meal and a little paternal interview. After several hours of wonderful interaction, my father announced rather shamelessly, "I would love for you to be my daughter-in-law."

Poor Despina. She had never even met me.

I know this sounds like a scene from a certain familiar Hollywood movie, but when we first laid eyes on each other, it was one of those love-at-first-sight kind of things. I knew she was the young woman God had been saving for me all these years. Six weeks into our courtship, we learned of an incredible coincidence. It seems that in 1977 my father was called on to see a young mother dying of cancer in a New York hospital. Dad prayed with her and provided spiritual comfort just days before her death. Twenty-six years later, Despina and I discovered that Dad had visited Despina's mother on her deathbed. Little nine-year-old Despina had lost her mother at a very tender age.

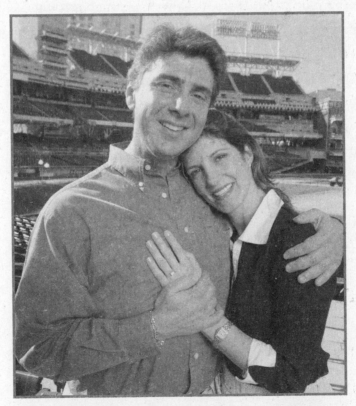

I like to tell people that I've gained 120 pounds since I married Despina on May 1, 2004. We did not get married at home plate at Petco Park in San Diego; instead we had a traditional big fat Greek wedding in my hometown.

Within seven weeks of our first date (there's that number seven again), I proposed to Despina on Thanksgiving Day (of course) with the entire family watching, including her father, whom I had flown out from New Jersey to join our family for Thanksgiving. I told you that Thanksgiving is my favorite holiday of the year.

So, this book has a happy ending. I got married, and now I don't have to listen to Dad or Mom saying, "Hey Nick, when are you going to find a girl and settle down?"

I found my girl, and she's beyond special to me. Love has brought a powerful motivation to stay healthy. I want to be around as long as possible with the one I cherish and with our children, if God grants us that desire.

You can say that I experienced a big fat Greek miracle in many ways, for which I am eternally grateful.

May God bless you,

—*Dr. Nick*

ABOUT THE AUTHORS

Nick Yphantides, M.D., is a family physician in Escondido, California, and a medical consultant to the nonprofit health-care agencies and the public health-care system regarding community health, foster children's health, child abuse prevention, domestic violence prevention, substance abuse prevention, personal health, fitness and promotion, and rural health care for the indigent.

The thirty-eight-year-old doctor is the son of a Greek immigrant and lived several years as a youth in Athens before returning to the United States. He graduated with honors from the University of California at San Diego School of Medicine in 1992, followed by training in family practice and preventative medicine. He is a former public elected official in San Diego County for the Palomar Pomerado Health Board. In May 2003, Dr. Nick was nominated to the Presidential Task Force/Commission on Nutrition, Fitness, and Public Health.

A much-in-demand speaker, Dr. Yphantides speaks on a variety of topics, including his personal weight-loss story. *My Big Fat Greek Diet* is his first book. He and his wife, Despina, make their home in Escondido.

Mike Yorkey is the author, coauthor, and collaborator of more than forty books, including several in the *Every Man's Battle* series and tennis star Michael Chang's autobiography, *Holding Serve*. He and his wife, Nicole, are the parents of two college-age children and live in Encinitas, California.

ACKNOWLEDGMENTS

The fingerprints and heartbeats of many precious people are on these pages. I highlight just a handful since I can't acknowledge everybody.

To my wife, Despina: The only thing missing in my life was you. I love you so much.

Dad: You were the most faithful and supportive travel companion—in life and on the trip—and the ultimate source of encouragement and guidance.

Mom: You have been the most selfless and enthusiastic cheerleader and a diligent source of faithful prayer support.

My brothers, Paul, John, and Phil: You have been my best friends and my "go-to" team for all matters of significance.

My sister, Pauline: You are my lovely sister and relentless supporter. I love your enthusiasm for life.

My sisters-in-law, Eleni, Heather, and Betsy: Thank you for completing the lives of my brothers.

My nephews and nieces, Coli, Sopie, Doey, Zankar, and Bernie (or better known as Nicole, Sophia, Joey, Alexander, and Bernice): You are the most cherished little lives to me. I love you and want to be around as long as I can for you.

My grandpa Pfaff: You were a pillar of support, inspiration, and companionship on the road and in life. Grandma would be so happy!

My entire extended family: May God's love keep us united.

Pastor Pat Kenney: You were the most consistent and diligent phone encourager.

Toni Hock and Mark Searle: You were generous and enthusiastic coordinators of my initial Web site, which was such a source of accountability to me and inspiration to others.

Brian Mavis: Thank you for being a dreamer who took the Web site up a notch.

Dr. Donald Miller: You were my baseball buddy and superb master planner for my trip.

Jose "Chuy" Escobedo and Mike Grant: You were my homeys on the road.

Kurt Varrichio: You were my personal Ticketmaster.

John Berhman, Jeff Frank, and Ed Lenderman: Your newspaper articles and TV features helped me put it all on the line right from the start. Thanks for telling San Diego about what this guy was up to.

Dr. Jim Schultz: Thank you for allowing my crazy idea to become a reality. By taking over my job at the Escondido Community Health Center, with Phil's help, you launched me off undistracted.

Brad Wiscons: The inspiration you were to me with your own 130-pound weight loss came at a very strategic time. Between us, we've lost 400 pounds. Let's never find them again.

The authors of 5,623 personal e-mails received during my eight-month trip: Your words of encouragement came at the right time and just kept coming.

The Chen, Vargas, and Kreopolidies families: Thank you for trusting me enough to leave the keys under the mat while you were away.

New York Yankee Scott Brosius: You provided what remains one of my most euphoric moments when you hit a home run in the bottom of the ninth inning in Game 5 of the World Series at 12:47 a.m. on November 2, 2001. Miracles do happen!

Joshua Chen: You were my youngest and most wide-eyed game companion.

Dave Biebel: Thank you for being the first one with publishing experience to seriously get me thinking about putting my story into a book form.

My coauthor, Mike Yorkey: You have done an amazing job in capturing the voice of my heart. Thank you so much.

My agent, Chip McGregor, and the Alive Communications staff: Thank you for your diligent representation.

Brian Hampton and everyone at Thomas Nelson: Thanks for your faith in me and for your sincere enthusiasm.

The Lord God Almighty: For every good thing I have in my life, I thank You. Words cannot capture Your love for me. "I can do all things through Christ who strengthens me" (Phil. 4:13 NKJV).

CONTACT INFORMATION

Dr. Nick Yphantides is available for
speaking engagements and media appearances.
If you would like to contact Dr. Nick Yphantides or purchase
autographed copies of this book, please go to his Web site at
www.healthsteward.com or call 1-877-DRNICK7 (1-877-376-4257).
Otherwise, you can write to:
Dr. Nick Yphantides
P.O. Box 1714
Escondido, CA 92033

DR. NICK'S STADIUM TOUR

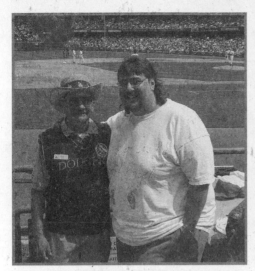

Dodger Stadium, Los Angeles Dodgers—467 pounds

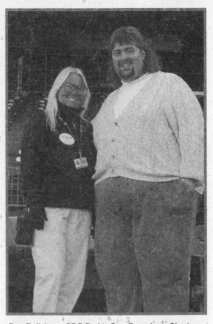

Pac Bell (now SBC Park), San Francisco Giants—460 pounds

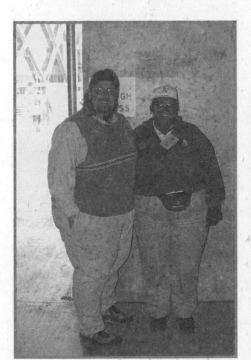

Network Associates Coliseum, Oakland A's—452 pounds

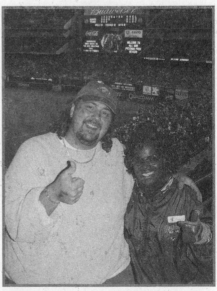

Qualcomm (they now play at Petco), San Diego Padres—448 pounds

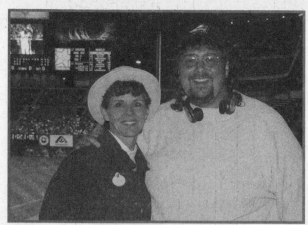

Angel Stadium, Anaheim Angels—
439 pounds

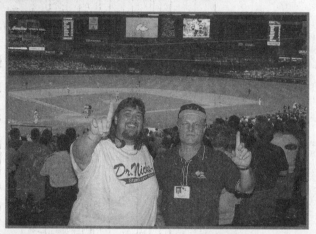

Bank One Ballpark, Arizona Diamondbacks —432 pounds

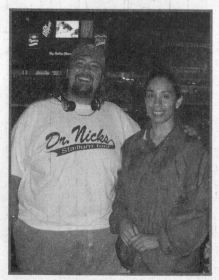

Ameriquest Field, Texas Rangers—416 pounds

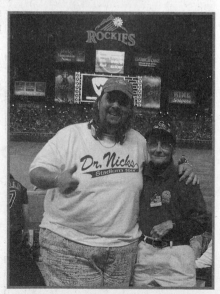

Coors Field, Colorado Rockies—410 pounds

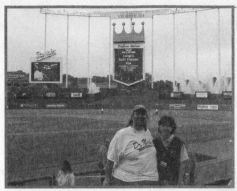

Kauffman Stadium, Kansas City Royals—
400 pounds

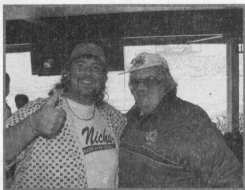

Fenway Park, Boston Red Sox—392 pounds

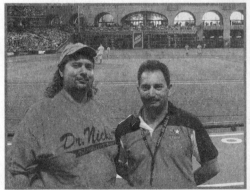

Enron (now Minute Maid Park), Houston Astros—
385 pounds

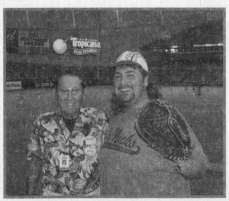

Tropicana Field, Tampa Bay Devil Rays—
377 pounds

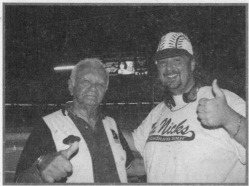

Pro Player Stadium, Florida Marlins—
374 pounds

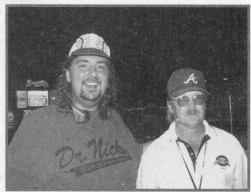

Turner Field, Atlanta Braves—370 pounds

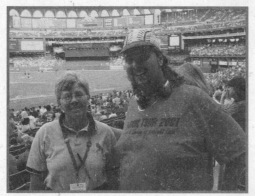

Busch Stadium, St. Louis Cardinals—367 pounds

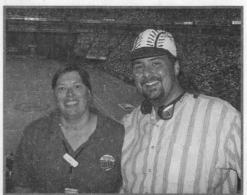

The Metrodome, Minnesota Twins—
364 pounds

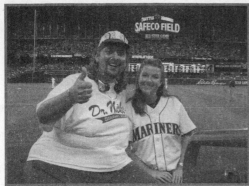

Safeco, Seattle Mariners—356 pounds

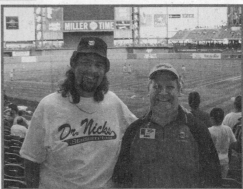

Miller Park, Milwaukee Brewers—345 pounds

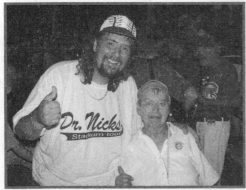

Wrigley Field, Chicago Cubs—337 pounds

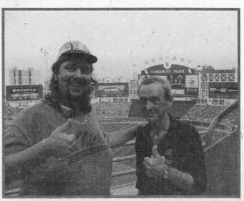

U.S. Cellular Field, Chicago White Sox—
335 pounds

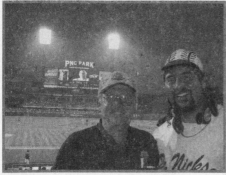

PNC Park, Pittsburgh Pirates—330 pounds

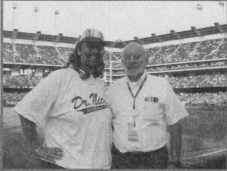

Jacobs Field, Cleveland Indians—325 pounds

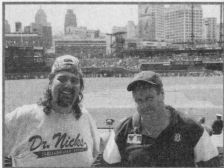

Comerica Park, Detroit Tigers—323 pounds

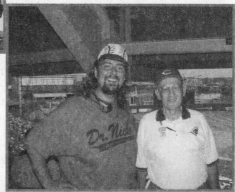

Cinergy (since demolished), Cincinnati Reds—320 pounds

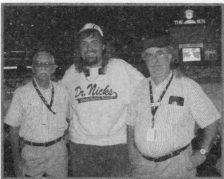

Oriole Park at Camden Yards, Baltimore Orioles—316 pounds

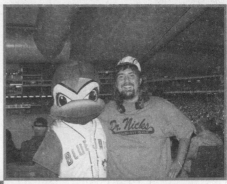

SkyDome, Toronto Blue Jays—313 pounds

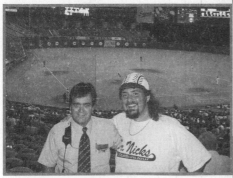

Olympic Stadium, Montreal Expos—312 pounds

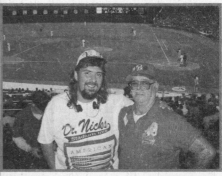

Veterans Stadium (since demolished), Philadelphia Phillies—298 pounds

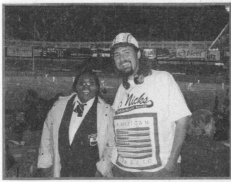

Yankee Stadium, New York Yankees—286 pounds

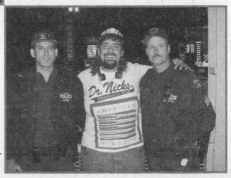

Shea Stadium, New York Mets—279 pounds